Critical Ca

Critical Care Physiology

Robert H. Bartlett, M.D.
Professor of Surgery and Director of Surgical Critical Care Program,
University of Michigan Medical School, Ann Arbor, Michigan

Scholarly Publishing Office, University of Michigan Library   Ann Arbor

Published in 2010 by The Scholarly Publishing Office
University of Michigan University Library

© 1996 Robert H. Bartlett

This edition is reprinted from the 1996 Little, Brown and Company edition by arrangement with Robert H. Bartlett

This work is licensed under a Creative Commons Attribution Non-Commercial 3.0 Unported License. License details are available at http://creativecommons.org/licenses/by-nc/3.0/

ISBN 978-1-60785-207-0

Contents

Preface vii

1. Oxygen Kinetics: Integrating Hemodynamic, Respiratory, and Metabolic Physiology 1
2. Blood Volume and Hemodynamics 24
3. Respiratory Physiology and Pathophysiology 48
4. Metabolism and Nutrition 101
5. Renal Physiology and Pathophysiology 134
6. Fluids and Electrolytes 155
7. Nervous System 176
8. Host Defenses 183

   Appendix 213

   Index 233

Preface

Fat medical textbooks are often accompanied by a pudgy, pocket-sized, small print, prose synopsis for instant reference by the student, resident, or practitioner. *Critical Care Physiology*, as the companion piece to *The Michigan Critical Care Handbook*, represents the opposite. *Critical Care Physiology* provides the explanations, references, methods, and other supportive information to flesh out the essentials presented in the handbook. *The Michigan Critical Care Handbook* is a slim, pocket reference that contains only graphs, charts, tables, and algorithms that are essential for the management of critically ill patients. The handbook contains no prose, procedures, or discussion, and it assumes a basic knowledge of pathophysiology.

Critical Care Physiology is limited to discussion of four organ systems (cardiovascular, respiratory, renal, and neurologic) and four topics in integrative physiology (oxygen kinetics, fluids and electrolytes, host defenses, and metabolism and nutrition). The focus is specifically on monitoring and management. A basic knowledge of anatomy, normal physiology, and general medicine is assumed. ICU procedures, pharmacology, basic bioengineering, and ICU devices and artificial organs are mentioned briefly; the references list sources of more complete descriptions.

The topics are presented as background in support of information for *The Michigan Critical Care Handbook* in a format modeled generally after the American Physiological Society's scholarly and encyclopedic *Handbook of Physiology*. This format includes the assumption of appropriate basic knowledge; selected topics discussed in depth; methods of measurement; classic graphs, charts, and tables from the literature; minimum discussion; and concise summary.

Unlike the *Handbook of Physiology*, the facts presented, the interpretations, and the recommendations are the selections and opinions of a single author. Although there are surely more qualified experts on each topic, this presumptuous effort is justified by the fact that whole patient care requires an integrated approach favoring, for example, neither the lungs nor the kidneys, neither the preload nor the afterload. Critical care often requires decisions based on risk and benefits, observation, and experience. In this book dogmatic recommendations are based primarily on risks and benefits observed by the author over a period of 30 years. Because of this, many of the opinions and diagrams are based on our own published research, without apology.

Both *Critical Care Physiology* and *The Michigan Critical Care Handbook* are intentionally simplified and dogmatic. The methods of monitoring and management described here will be applicable to 95% of critical patient care. The justification for axioms and treatment recommendations is included in the text, but no attempt is made to include all the pertinent references or contrasting theories. Several excellent, exhaustive texts of critical care extensively review such literature. *The Michigan Critical Care Handbook* is intended for practical use at the bedside; therefore, the emphasis is entirely on physiology, pathophysiology, and macrophysiologic management. Intracellular, subcellular, and molecular phenomena are discussed only as they relate specifically to whole organ and whole patient care. This should not minimize the importance of molecular biology in critical illness; other excellent textbooks, symposia, and entire journals are devoted solely to those topics.

Critical Care Physiology and *The Michigan Critical Care Handbook* focus on visual presentations and algorithms based on the assumption that the physiology and pathophysiology of critical illness are best learned and described through graphic presentation. Most of the graphs, figures, and tables in the handbook are original drawings by the author adapted from dozens of standard sources. These include the oxyhemoglobin dissociation curves, Frank-Starling cardiac function curve, pulmonary compliance curves, and others. The figures in *The Michigan Critical Care Handbook* were selected to be the most descriptive and most useful for quick reference in critical care. Many of the other classic presentations of critical care physiology are presented as figures in *Critical Care Physiology*. A single graph of the bicarbonate buffer system, for example, is presented in the handbook while several classic and common variations on the graph are presented in this text.

All of intensive care is based on measurement, and precise measurement of physiologic variables makes intensive care possible. In this book and in clinical practice, however, precise measurement is not necessary. While it is not important to measure the arterial blood pressure to 3 decimal places, not even to single units, it *is* important to know the blood pressure within about 5% of the precise value. The same is true of blood gases, chemical measurements, and calculated descriptors such as shunt fraction or vascular resistance. Consequently, numerical values in this book are usually expressed as round numbers, which are easy to remember, rather than precisely accurate numbers. As an example, normal arterial oxygen content is described as 20 cc/dL, although the precise value is closer to 20.5. Normal cardiac index is identified in graphs and tables as 3 $L/m^2/min$, although the accurate number is 3.2. Physiologic purists will note that my selection of important constants is, at times, arbitrary and that conventional notation is sometimes ignored. For example, the amount of oxygen that 1 gm of hemoglobin can bind is given as 1.36 cc, and the solubility coefficient for oxygen is given as .003 cc/mm Hg/dL. Many measurements are expressed in terms that make the most sense in teaching the concepts, rather than in proper arithmetic form.

In the example just given, oxygen solubility is expressed as cc of oxygen per unit of pressure per unit of volume, rather than k × mm Hg^{-1} × dL. Some new shorthand is invented, particularly ⓜ to represent "per square meter per minute" and Ⓝ to indicate the normal value on charts and graphs.

Although measuring is central to management of the critically ill patient, many of the values are relatively useless without normalizing the values to the size of the patient. For example, a cardiac output of 4 L/min may represent shock for a large muscular man and luxuriant perfusion for a little old lady. Hemodynamic variables are usually normalized to body surface area—an unwieldy combination of height and weight that requires a table of values for reference. Drug doses and metabolic variables are usually normalized to kilogram of body weight without regard to relative amounts of fat, water, or lean body mass. Although both of these methods of normalizing are imperfect, they are necessary, particularly when writing a book intended to describe pathophysiology for all adults. Another common approach is to describe physiologic variables as they would be found in a typical 70 kg, lean, healthy, young man. All of these methods of normalization and example are used in this book.

This two volume set is dual-purpose: *The Michigan Critical Care Handbook* offers concise, quick-reference graphs and tables of crucial information, while *Critical Care Physiology* provides further explanation and expansion for the interested reader. Comments, suggestions, and corrections are welcomed by the author.

R.H.B.

Critical Care Physiology

Notice. The indications for and dosages of all drugs in this book have been recommended in the medical literature and conform to the practices of the general medical community. The medications described do not necessarily have specific approval by the Food and Drug Administration for use in the diseases and dosages for which they are recommended. The package insert for each drug should be consulted for use and dosage as approved by the FDA. Because standards for usage change, it is advisable to keep abreast of revised recommendations, particularly those concerning drugs.

1

Oxygen Kinetics:
Integrating Hemodynamic, Respiratory, and Metabolic Physiology

Monitoring and management of critically ill patients is an exercise in applied physiology and pharmacology made possible through applied bioengineering. The intensive care unit affords the possibility to monitor a wide variety of physiologic variables continuously and to use that information to prevent and treat organ failure. Central to the intelligent use of this information is an understanding of homeostatic physiology: integrated cardiac, respiratory, and metabolic physiology (oxygen kinetics); hemodynamics; respiratory physiology; nutrition and metabolism; renal pathophysiology; fluids and electrolytes; and host defenses (Figure 1-1).

Oxygen Consumption

The fire of life is maintained by the continuous oxidation of chemical substrates, consuming oxygen and producing carbon dioxide in the process. The oxygen consumed in this process of metabolism is expressed as the volume of oxygen consumed per minute ($\dot{V}O_2$). $\dot{V}O_2$ is normally 100 to 120 cc/m^2/min, or 200 cc/min for a typical adult. The resting $\dot{V}O_2$ is a function of the metabolizing body cell mass, with fine-tuning control provided by the levels of thyroid and catecholamine hormones and governed by a poorly understood metabolic controller in the hypothalamus. $\dot{V}O_2$ decreases under conditions of hypothermia, paralysis, and hypothyroidism. It increases during exercise or other muscular activity, hyperthermia, profound hypothalamic injury, hyperthyroidism, and a rise in the catecholamine level, and in the presence of inflammatory mediators, particularly the interleukin cytokines. The metabolism that occurs in different organs proceeds at different rates depending on the cell mass and cellular activity, so systemic $\dot{V}O_2$ is affected to some extent by changes in regional blood flow. Under steady-state conditions, the amount of oxygen consumed in the process of systemic

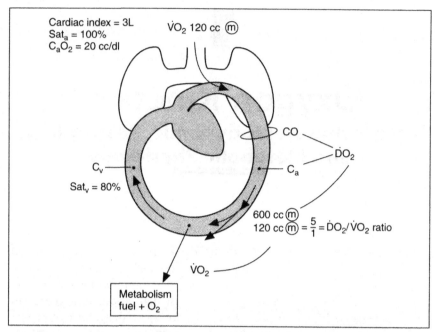

FIGURE 1-1. Oxygen kinetics. Oxygen delivery ($\dot{D}O_2$) is the product of cardiac output (CO) times the arterial oxygen content (C_a). Oxygen delivery is normally four to five times oxygen consumption ($\dot{V}O_2$). (C_v = venous oxygen content; ⓜ = /min/m^2; Sat_a = arterial saturation; Sat_v = venous saturation.)

metabolism is exactly equal to the amount of oxygen taken up in the pulmonary capillaries by means of the airway (Fick's axiom). This is true regardless of the status of pulmonary function or dysfunction, so we measure $\dot{V}O_2$ across the lung and assume that this is exactly the amount consumed in systemic metabolism. The efficiency of oxygen uptake across the lung is controlled by the match between perfusion and inflation of alveolar units. As long as normally perfused alveoli are inflated and contain gas with an oxygen concentration of 20% or higher, the perfusate blood is fully oxygenated.

Measurements of $\dot{V}O_2$

Assuming Fick's axiom to be correct, $\dot{V}O_2$ during metabolism in body tissues can be measured in three ways: (1) closed-circuit rebreathing volumetric spirometry, (2) open-circuit mixed expired gas analysis; or (3) calculation of arteriovenous oxygen content difference times cardiac output. Closed-circuit rebreathing volumetric spirometry is the gold standard method for measuring $\dot{V}O_2$. The subject breathes into and out of a low-resistance spirometer equipped with a CO_2 absorber. As oxygen is absorbed the volume loss in

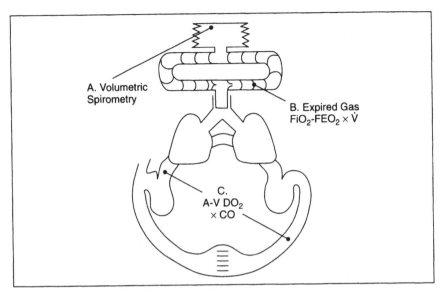

FIGURE 1-2. Three methods of measuring oxygen consumption: closed-circuit–rebreathing volumetric spirometry **A.**, mixed expired gas analysis **B.**, and the Fick equation **C.** (A-V DO_2 = arteriovenous oxygen content difference; CO = cardiac output; FEO_2 = fraction of expired oxygen; $\dot{V}$ = volume)

the closed system can be measured. $\dot{V}O_2$ is measured over 5 to 10 minutes and averaged, and the results are reported as the oxygen consumed per minute after conversion from ATPS (ambient temperature and pressure, saturated) to STPD (standard temperature and pressure, day). Because it is a direct volumetric measurement, any small leak in the system will result in major errors in measurement; therefore this technique cannot be used in a patient with a bronchopleural cutaneous fistula, for example. Complete closure at the mouth and nose is essential. The technique is excellent for intubated patients whose airway is totally controlled (Figure 1-2).

The second method of measuring $\dot{V}O_2$ is by measuring the concentration of oxygen in inspired and expired gas and multiplying the difference times the minute volume. This method requires precise measurement of oxygen concentration in mixed expired gas, precise measurement of exhaled minute volume, and precise measurement (or assumption) of inspired oxygen concentration. Because the inspired oxygen concentration is known and constant when the subject is breathing air, mixed expired gas analysis is ideally suited for air-breathing patients, during physiologic studies of the effects of exercise, for example. For the same reason this technique is not well suited for use in patients who require supplemental inspired oxygen because a very small error in maintaining the constancy or measuring the concentration of inspired oxygen (50.5% versus 51%, for example) can result in large errors in $\dot{V}O_2$ calculation. The accuracy of this technique can also be affected by the fact that the breath-by-breath volume of inspired gas versus expired gas can be slightly different because the amount of CO_2 exhaled may not be exactly equal to the amount of oxygen absorbed from each breath. If the ratio of CO_2 produced to oxygen consumed (the respiratory quotient [RQ]) is 1.0, then the inhaled and exhaled volumes will be exactly equal; hence if only the exhaled volume is measured, this exactly predicts the inspired volume. However, if the patient is hyperventilating and CO_2 production ($\dot{V}CO_2$) exceeds $\dot{V}O_2$, or if the patient is primarily metabolizing fat and the RQ is 0.7, then the exhaled volume is not exactly equal to the inspired volume from which oxygen was consumed. This problem can be dealt with in one of three ways: (1) by assuming a constant RQ of 0.8; (2) by measuring inspired and expired nitrogen concentrations and correcting minute ventilation, assuming that the amount of nitrogen inspired and expired per minute is exactly equal; or (3) by assuming the RQ is 1.0 and ignoring the artifact. In practice the third option is usually followed because the error associated with not correcting for RQ is small. Values are measured under ATPS conditions and converted to STPD. When using mixed expired gas analysis, both the $\dot{V}CO_2$ and $\dot{V}O_2$ are measured, and the RQ is calculated. The RQ should be close to 1.0 to prove that a steady state without hyperventilation existed during the period of measurement (or the RQ should correspond to the physiologic conditions, such as 0.7 during starvation).

The third method of $\dot{V}O_2$ measurement is a variation of the Fick equation and consists in the multiplication of the arteriovenous oxygen content difference ($AVDO_2$) times the cardiac output measured by thermal or indicator dilution. This method requires accurate measurement of oxygen content in both arterial and mixed venous blood; hence it is possible to use it only in patients who have a pulmonary artery catheter in place. Because the measurement of indicator dilution cardiac output is accurate to within 5% at best and the measurement of arterial and venous oxygen content is accurate to within 5%, the range of error of the $\dot{V}O_2$ calculation using this method is within 10% at best. Consequently this method is the least accurate and is used only for rough estimates of $\dot{V}O_2$ or in circumstances such as large air leaks in which closed-circuit or mixed expired gas analysis methods cannot be used. Because the constants used for calculating oxygen content from the partial pressure of oxygen (PO_2) and saturation are expressed in STPD units, further conversion is not necessary. Whatever method is used to measure $\dot{V}O_2$, it is important to remember that normal values and calculations are always based on STPD conditions. Conversion from ATPS to STPD may decrease the volume by 15% to 20%, so careful attention to accurate measurement of temperature and humidity is important.

There are several simple methods for checking the accuracy of $\dot{V}O_2$ measurements. The RQ should be close to 1.0, or correspond to expected physiologic variations, as already mentioned. Steady state should be assured by checking the $\dot{V}O_2$ measurements each minute during a 5- or 10-minute collection period. Minute-to-minute variations should be less than 5%. The

$\dot{V}O_2$ should correspond to the observed physiologic state. For example, if a normothermic, sedated patient at rest has a $\dot{V}O_2$ 50% greater than the normal levels, there is probably either a leak in the system or an error in calculation. This can be checked further by calculating the ventilation equivalent for oxygen or CO_2. Under most conditions the minute ventilation will be 2.5 to 4 liters for each 100 cc of oxygen consumed or CO_2 produced. If the ventilation equivalent for oxygen or CO_2 is outside this range, an error in measurement is likely. The $\dot{V}O_2$ and $\dot{V}CO_2$ can be measured very simply in mechanically ventilated patients by accurately measuring the minute ventilation and collecting samples of mixed inspired and mixed expired gas, then measuring oxygen and CO_2 concentration in any standard blood gas machine. If all the variables and potential errors mentioned are accounted for, this method of analysis yields very accurate information at little cost. There are also very expensive "metabolic carts" that do essentially the same thing.

Once the $\dot{V}O_2$ is accurately measured, it is used in three ways: (1) to determine whether the patient is hypermetabolic or hypometabolic; (2) to determine and regulate the relationship between oxygen delivery ($\dot{D}O_2$) and $\dot{V}O_2$; and (3) to calculate the caloric expenditure of metabolism. Normal $\dot{V}O_2$ is 100 to 120 $cc/m^2/min$, or 3 to 5 cc $O_2/kg/min$. A $\dot{V}O_2$ above this range in a resting, nonexercising subject indicates the presence of active inflammation, usually infection. Changes in metabolism are followed by compensatory changes in $\dot{D}O_2$ to maintain a $\dot{D}O_2$ ratio of 5:1. To determine whether $\dot{D}O_2$ is adequate, inadequate, or excessive, it is necessary to know both the $\dot{D}O_2$ and $\dot{V}O_2$. This is discussed in detail in the next section. $\dot{V}O_2$ measurement can be converted to the caloric equivalent of metabolic substrate for purposes of nutritional planning by doing calculations known as *indirect calorimetry*. This is discussed in detail in Chapter 4, but in brief, 5 kcal worth of substrate is metabolized for each liter of oxygen consumed.

Oxygen Delivery

Oxygen is delivered from the lung to the systemic tissues by means of the blood. The amount of oxygen delivered to peripheral tissues is the product of the oxygen content in arterial blood times the cardiac output (Figure 1-3).

Normally the oxygen content of arterial blood (CaO_2) is 20 cc/dL, and the normal cardiac index (CI) is 3.2 $L/m^2/min$ (5 L/min for a typical adult). Therefore the normal $\dot{D}O_2$ is 20 cc/dL × 50 dL/min = 1000 cc/min (Figure 1-4).

Although oxygen content is the most important measurement of oxygen in blood, PO_2 and oxyhemoglobin saturation are most commonly measured in the ICU, hence it is necessary to convert among these measurements. Each gram of hemoglobin can bind 1.36 cc of oxygen. If the hemoglobin of the blood is normal (15 g/dL) and the hemoglobin is 100% saturated, the amount of oxygen bound to hemoglobin is 20.4 cc/dL. In addition, a small amount of oxygen is physically dissolved in the water that makes up plasma and red

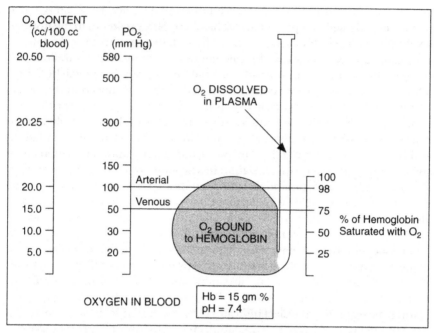

FIGURE 1-3. Schematic representation of the distribution of oxygen in blood. The amount of oxygen bound to hemoglobin (*Hb*) is represented in the flask, in equilibrium with the amount of oxygen dissolved in plasma, represented as the small graduated cylinder. (From: Bartlett RH. Post traumatic pulmonary insufficiency. In: Cooper P, Nyhus L, eds. Surgery Annual, 1971. New York: Appleton-Century-Crofts, 1971.)

blood cells. The solubility coefficient for oxygen is 0.0031 cc/mm Hg/dL, and therefore the amount of oxygen dissolved in 1 dL of blood at a P_{O_2} of 100 mm Hg is 0.3 cc, making the oxygen content of normal arterial blood 20.4 + 0.3 = 20.7 cc/dL, which for convenience sake is rounded off to 20 cc/dL. Using the same arithmetic, the oxygen content of venous blood (CvO_2) is 16 cc/dL, hence the normal $AVDO_2$ is 4 cc of O_2/dL. The relationship among P_{O_2}, saturation, and oxygen content for different concentrations of hemoglobin is shown in Figures 1-3 and 1-4. Notice that the P_{O_2} and saturation are the same for anemic arterial and venous blood even though the oxygen content is severely decreased.

Measuring Oxygen in Blood

The most common method of measuring the amount of oxygen in blood is to measure the partial pressure of oxygen (P_{O_2}) in a blood gas machine. Blood gas machines use a system referred to as the Clark electrode, which

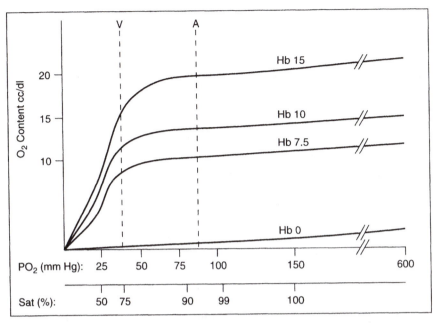

FIGURE 1-4. The amount of oxygen in blood can be expressed as the oxygen content, P_{O_2}, or saturation of hemoglobin (*SAT*). In this figure all three measurements are applied to blood ranging from normal (hemoglobin, 15 g/dL) to anemia (hemoglobin, 7.5 g/dL) to plasma (hemoglobin, 0). The typical values for normal arterial (A) and venous (V) blood are shown. Notice that P_{O_2} and saturation are normal in anemic blood even though the oxygen content is severely decreased.

was developed by Leland Clark more than thirty years ago. The underlying principle of the Clark electrode is that the flow of electrical current in a platinum wire is proportionate to the concentration of oxygen. The Clark P_{O_2} electrode includes a platinum cathode and a silver chloride anode held in a potassium chloride solution, encased in glass, and covered with a plastic membrane that is permeable to oxygen. When a gas or fluid containing oxygen is applied to the membrane and allowed to come into equilibrium, the resulting current flow can be used to determine the oxygen concentration in the sample when the entire device has been calibrated against known standards. P_{O_2} values measured by the Clark electrode are accurate to $\pm 1\%$.

The oxyhemoglobin saturation is measured with an infrared spectrophotometer. In this method, infrared light with two or three specific wavelengths is shone into the blood sample and the amount of reflected light is measured. Wavelengths are chosen to represent a point at which reduced and oxygenated hemoglobin have the same absorbance (the reference point) and another wavelength at which the absorbance of reduced and oxygenated hemoglobin is widely divergent. Accuracy over the full range of absorbance can be further ensured by using a third or fourth wavelength. The spectrophotometer can be calibrated against an internal standard and does not require separate blood or fluid calibration; however, there is a tendency for drift to occur in most spectrophotometers, so recalibration should be done fairly frequently. The spectrophotometer is used to measure the amount of saturation basically by examining the color of the reflected light. The total amount of hemoglobin can be measured by examining the intensity of reflected light. In addition, by using other infrared wavelengths the amount of carboxyhemoglobin or methemoglobin can also be measured. Spectrophotometers that make these measurements are referred to as *oximeters*.

Oximeters are available that make use of fiberoptic technology to continuously measure the saturation in arterial or venous blood, and this involves the use of fiberoptic-equipped catheters attached to external spectrophotometers. These devices have proved to be exceptionally valuable for critical care, particularly when used for continuous mixed venous oximetry. Another very useful variation on the continuous oximeter is the application of infrared light to capillary beds in the fingers, toes, or earlobes. Infrared light applied in this fashion shows considerable variation in absorption, ranging from that of arterial to that of venous blood in the capillaries. If the device is programmed with a microchip to display only the highest levels of saturation that occur during systole when arterial blood surges into the capillaries, it can provide a reasonable estimate of arterial blood saturation. Devices of this type are referred to as *pulse oximeters,* and the value displayed is commonly referred to as SpO_2. Although any factor that minimizes peripheral perfusion can cause artifacts in SpO_2 measurement, this monitoring technique is still very valuable for detecting extreme hypoxia or poor peripheral blood flow and for making gross adjustments in the mechanical ventilator setting or the amount of supplemental oxygen administered. The range of error of the best blood oximeters is $\pm 2\%$, and the range of error of pulse oximeters versus the actual arterial blood saturation values is $\pm 5\%$. It is important to note that blood saturation can be calculated based on Po_2, pH, and temperature if all three variables are known. When oxyhemoglobin saturation is calculated in this fashion, it is assumed that the oxyhemoglobin dissociation curve is normal, which is often not the case in critically ill patients. Consequently, the oxyhemoglobin saturations measured on many blood gas machines are simply calculations and may be considerably in error. If saturation is used to calculate the oxygen content or to adjust mechanical ventilators or oxygen treatment, the saturation should be measured directly with oximeter rather than calculated from the Po_2.

The direct measurement of oxygen content is by far the most important way of determining the amount of oxygen in blood but is the most difficult and therefore the most rarely performed. The classic method for measuring oxygen content is to displace all the oxygen from a precisely measured aliquot of blood using a combination of vacuum forces and strong reducing agents. The gas thus liberated includes oxygen, CO_2, and nitrogen. The total volume of gas is measured; the CO_2 and then the oxygen are selectively removed; and the volume of each can then be determined by subtraction. This method is extremely tedious, time-consuming, and operator dependent. It is known as the *Van Slyke method*, with variations designed and described by Sholander, Natelson, and others. The range of error when it is performed by a very experienced operator is ±3%. Direct measurement of oxygen content measured in this fashion is almost never utilized in modern critical care medicine. A second method for directly measuring oxygen content is the fuel cell system. In this system a precisely measured aliquot of blood is exposed to a vacuum force; oxygen is then released and consumed in an oxidative process, which generates an electrical signal exactly proportional to the amount of oxygen liberated from the blood. The original fuel cell system was produced by Lexington Instruments and called the *Lex-O-Con*. Although the fuel cell method is much easier and as accurate as the Van Slyke method, it is still difficult to perform, operator dependent, and rarely utilized. Because of these difficulties, even though oxygen content is by far the most important determination of the amount of oxygen in blood, it is almost always calculated from other measurements rather than measured directly. It is calculated by measuring the total hemoglobin level in grams per deciliter, the amount of hemoglobin that has oxygen bound to it using an oximeter and measuring the P_{O_2} of oxygen dissolved in plasma. These quantities are converted into cubic centimeters of oxygen using the constants described earlier, with the final value reported as the oxygen content. The range of error in the P_{O_2}, hemoglobin, and saturation measurements is considerable; the oxygen contents derived in this fashion are accurate ±5%.

Estimating $\dot{D}_{O_2}$

Despite the range of error associated with all the various measurements just mentioned, it is still very valuable to calculate the $\dot{D}_{O_2}$ in critically ill patients. This is done by measuring the hemoglobin level and saturation, calculating the content (usually ignoring the dissolved fraction if the P_{O_2} is less than 100 mm Hg), and then multiplying the arterial oxygen content times the cardiac output. This calculation gives the oxygen delivery in cubic centimeters of oxygen per minute with a range of error of ±15%. All physiologic variables should be normalized to the patient's body size. By convention, $\dot{D}_{O_2}$ and $\dot{V}_{O_2}$ measurements are normalized to the body surface area. To accomplish this the arterial oxygen content is multiplied by the cardiac *index* to give the content in cubic centimeters per minute per square meter of body surface area. The normal value is 600 cc/O_2/m²/min. In the graph shown in Figure 1-5, $\dot{D}_{O_2}$ has been calculated and displayed for a wide range of hemoglobin levels and cardiac index values. The normal point is shown as a cardiac index of 3 L/m²/min and $\dot{D}_{O_2}$ of 600 cc/O_2/m²/min (Figure 1-5). Definitions and formulas related to oxygen kinetics are summarized in Table 1-1.

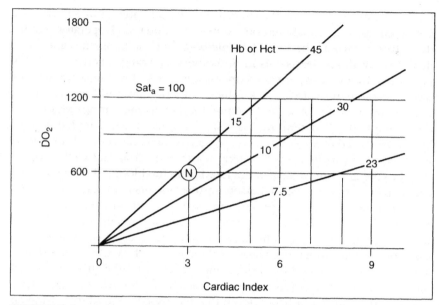

FIGURE 1-5. Estimating oxygen delivery. When the cardiac index and hemoglobin (*Hb*) level or hematocrit *Hct* is known, and if the arterial saturation (Sat_a) is close to 100%, the systemic oxygen delivery ($\dot{D}O_2$) can be quickly estimated using this graph.

TABLE 1-1. Oxygen Kinetics

Abbreviation	Definition	Normal value
CaO_2	Oxygen content, arterial	20 cc/dL
CvO_2	Oxygen content, venous	16 cc/dL
$AVDO_2$	Arteriovenous oxygen content difference	4 cc/dL
$\dot{D}O_2$	Oxygen delivery	600 cc/min/m²
$\dot{V}O_2$	Oxygen consumption	120 cc/min/m²
$\dot{V}CO_2$	CO_2 produced	100 cc/min/m²
REE	Resting energy expenditure	25 cal/kg/day
ⓜ	—	/min/m²

Oxygen Content = (Hb g/dL × % sat × 1.36 cc/g) + (PO_2 × 0.003 cc of O_2/mm Hg/dL)
Oxygen Delivery = CaO_2 × Cardiac index
Fick's axiom: O_2 consumed via lung = O_2 consumed in metabolism
CaO_2 or CvO_2 = Oxygen Content = cc of O_2/dL = O_2 bound to Hb + O_2 dissolved:
   O_2 bound to Hb = Hb g/dL × % sat × 1.36 cc of O_2/g,
   O_2 dissolved = PO_2 × 0.003 cc of O_2/mm Hg/dL
$AVDO_2 = CaO_2 - CvO_2$

Autoregulation to Maintain $\dot{D}o_2$

The relationships between $\dot{V}o_2$ and $\dot{D}o_2$ represent one of the most interesting autoregulation systems in homeostasis. First of all, if one of the three components of $\dot{D}o_2$ is abnormal, endogenous mechanisms are activated to regulate the other two until normal $\dot{D}o_2$ has been restored. These relationships are shown in Figures 1-6 and 1-7.

To compensate for acute hypoxia or acute anemia (Figure 1-6), cardiac output increases but only until normal $\dot{D}o_2$ is reestablished. In chronic hypoxia the red blood cell mass increases until the $\dot{D}o_2$ is normal at a normal cardiac output. This mechanism is triggered by secretion of erythropoietin from the kidney. In chronic anemia, cardiac output increases and remains increased. The mechanism primarily consists in a change in viscosity while the arterial tone remains constant. When cardiac output is decreased, there is no mechanism to induce superoxygenation or polycythemia. In this situation $\dot{V}o_2$ generally continues at the normal rate of metabolism and relatively more oxygen is extracted from the flowing blood, thus widening the $AVDO_2$ (see Figure 1-7).

The various combinations of these compensatory mechanisms ensures that adequate oxygen is supplied so that systemic metabolism can take place throughout a wide range of variations in $\dot{D}o_2$. If $\dot{D}o_2$ cannot be maintained at a level at least twice the $\dot{V}o_2$, an unstable state results, and this is described in the next sections.

Autoregulation for Changing $\dot{V}o_2$

When there is a change in the metabolic rate, there is a proportionate change in $\dot{D}o_2$, which occurs almost immediately and is mediated completely by a change in cardiac output. For example, when one goes from rest to mild exercise, $\dot{V}o_2$ doubles; this is followed promptly by an increase in cardiac output (Figure 1-8), thereby reestablishing the $\dot{D}o_2/\dot{V}o_2$ ratio at approximately 5 : 1. The mechanism responsible for mediating this change in cardiac output is not fully understood but probably involves a chemoreceptor on the venous side of the circulation and vasodilation in working muscles. This autoregulation occurs regardless of whether the change in $\dot{V}o_2$ is increased or decreased, and whether it is caused by fever (Figure 1-9), exercise, sepsis, catecholamines, or the presence of other mediators (see Figure 1-8).

Autoregulation for Changing $\dot{V}o_2$ with Exercise

As shown in Figure 1-8, conditions causing hypermetabolism in critically ill patients might increase the metabolic rate by 20%, 30%, 50%, or very rarely

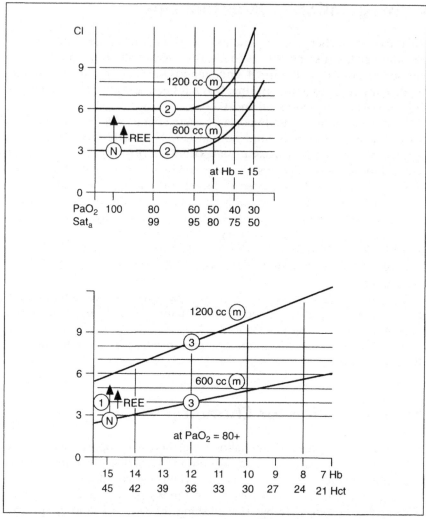

FIGURE 1-6. Oxygen delivery ($\dot{D}o_2$) is normally maintained at a level four to five times greater than oxygen consumption by changes in endogenous cardiac output. In this figure, typical changes in cardiac output to maintain normal $\dot{D}o_2$ in the presence of other variables are demonstrated. The relationships are shown for normal metabolism ($\dot{D}o_2$ = 600 cc/min/m²) and hypermetabolism ($\dot{D}o_2$ = 1200 c/min/m²). Line *1* shows the increase in cardiac index required for an increase in $\dot{V}o_2$ or energy expenditure. Line *2* shows the change in cardiac index required to maintain normal $\dot{D}o_2$ in the face of progressive hypoxia. Line *3* shows the change in the cardiac index required to maintain normal $\dot{D}o_2$ during progressive levels of anemia. (Hb = hemoglobin; Hct = hematocrit; Ⓜ = /min/m²; Ⓝ = normal; REE = resting energy expenditure; Sat_a = arterial saturation.)

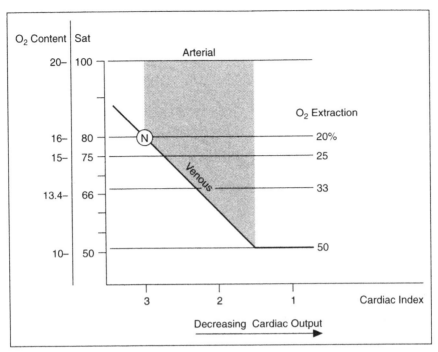

FIGURE 1-7. The shaded area shows compensation for decreasing cardiac output brought about by increasing the amount of oxygen extracted from each deciliter of flowing blood. Relationships are shown for normal metabolism. ($\dot{V}O_2$ = 120 cc/m^2/min). Normally only 20% of oxygen is extracted, leaving the venous blood 80% saturated. Increased extraction of oxygen can compensate for low blood flow without producing physiologic side effects until the ratio of delivery to consumption is below 2:1. At 2:1 ratio the venous blood is 50% saturated. (Ⓝ = normal, Sat = saturation.)

100% above the normal baseline rate. This change in metabolism is different from the changes associated with exercise, in which $\dot{V}O_2$ doubles with very mild exercise, such as walking. With vigorous exercise, $\dot{V}O_2$ increases by 10 to 20 times the normal rate. As in the setting of the critical care conditions described earlier, cardiac output increases as the metabolic rate accelerates to maintain the $\dot{D}O_2/\dot{V}O_2$ ratio at 5:1. When the cardiac output has reached its maximum, increased activity is further compensated for by increasing the peripheral extraction of oxygen to venous saturation levels as low as 20%. Maximal $\dot{V}O_2$ during exercise to the point of exhaustion is referred to in the exercise physiology literature as $\dot{V}O_2max$ and is the method by which being "in shape" is measured. It is somewhat of a misnomer, however, because the limiting factor is not the maximal amount of oxygen consumed but rather the maximal cardiac output that can be generated in response to an elevated $\dot{V}O_2$.

14 Critical Care Physiology

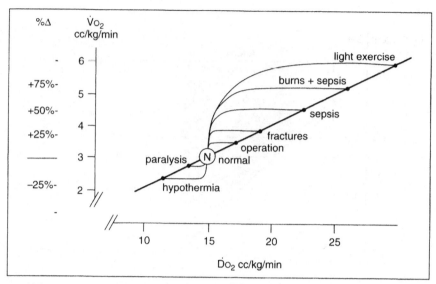

FIGURE 1-8. Change in $\dot{V}O_2$, and compensatory change in $\dot{D}O_2$, related to typical conditions that affect critically ill patients. (Ⓝ = normal.)

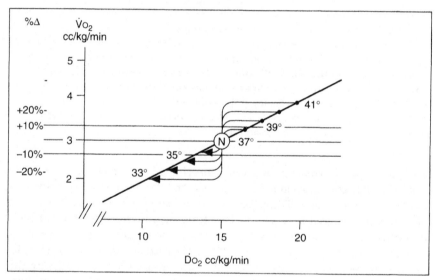

FIGURE 1-9. Change in $\dot{V}O_2$, and compensatory change in $\dot{D}O_2$, related to a change in body temperature. (Ⓝ = normal.)

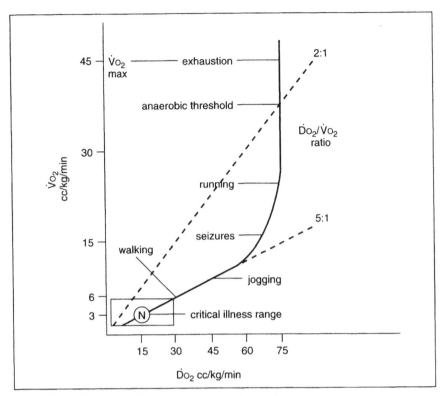

FIGURE 1-10. $\dot{V}O_2$ and cardiac output compensation during exercise compared with conditions encountered in critical illness. In this example the maximum cardiac output is five times the resting level.

In a trained runner, the $\dot{V}O_2$ at rest is 0.1 L/m²/min and the $\dot{V}O_2$max might be 20 L/m²/min. In a frail patients with cardiac disease, the resting $\dot{V}O_2$ might be 0.1 L/m²/min and the $\dot{V}O_2$max, 0.3 L/m²/min. These relationships are shown in Figure 1-10.

Autoregulation for Changing $\dot{D}O_2$

A primary change in $\dot{D}O_2$ is *not* followed by any change in $\dot{V}O_2$, nor would we expect the $\dot{V}O_2$ to change because systemic $\dot{D}O_2$ is not among the controllers of metabolism. However, it is obvious that $\dot{V}O_2$ cannot exceed $\dot{D}O_2$, and if $\dot{D}O_2$ did decrease below the $\dot{V}O_2$, $\dot{V}O_2$ would become supply dependent. In theory this would occur when the $\dot{D}O_2/\dot{V}O_2$ ratio is below 1:1. In actuality, however, the supply dependency of $\dot{V}O_2$ occurs when the $\dot{D}O_2$ decreases to below twice the $\dot{V}O_2$, that is, supply dependency occurs when the ratio of $\dot{D}O_2$ to $\dot{V}O_2$ is less than 2:1. This relationship is shown in Figure 1-11, which demonstrates the biphasic nature of the $\dot{V}O_2/\dot{D}O_2$ relationship.

16 Critical Care Physiology

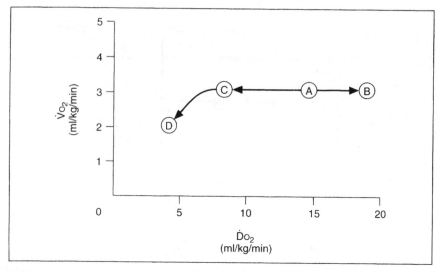

FIGURE 1-11. The normal relationship between $\dot{V}O_2$ and $\dot{D}O_2$. The normal point (A) is shown as $\dot{V}O_2$ 120 cc/m²/min and $\dot{D}O_2$ 600 cc/m²/min. If $\dot{D}O_2$ is increased by transfusion (B), $\dot{V}O_2$ remains constant. If $\dot{D}O_2$ is progressively decreased (A to C), $\dot{V}O_2$ remains constant until the ratio of $\dot{D}O_2/\dot{V}O_2$ falls below 2:1 (C to D).

When a state of supply dependency exists, anaerobic metabolism occurs, an oxygen debt develops, hemodynamic instability eventuates, and if the situation lasts long enough, progressive organ failure occurs and the patient can be said to be in a state of circulatory, ischemic, or hypoxic shock. The same relationships exist when the $\dot{V}O_2$ is elevated in the setting of hypermetabolism, as shown in Figure 1-12.

Supply dependency arises during hypermetabolism whenever the $\dot{D}O_2/\dot{V}O_2$ ratio is less than 2:1, although this occurs at a higher level of actual $\dot{D}O_2$ during hypermetabolism than it does during normal metabolism. The primary goal of intensive care management is to estimate or determine the $\dot{V}O_2$ and $\dot{D}O_2$, to maintain the patient near the normal ratio of 5:1, and if oxygen delivery fails, to intervene before the ratio reaches the critically low level of approximately 2:1 (Figure 1-13).

Arterial and Venous Saturation Monitoring

The relationship between $\dot{D}O_2$ and $\dot{V}O_2$ is reflected by the amount of oxygen in venous blood. Under normal conditions in an average adult, $\dot{D}O_2$ is 1,000 cc/min and $\dot{V}O_2$ is 200 cc/min. The amount of oxygen extracted is 20% of that delivered, and 80% of the oxygen is still present in venous blood returning to the heart. Usually the arterial blood is fully saturated, and under normal

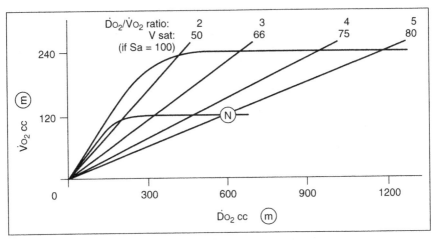

FIGURE 1-12. $\dot{D}O_2/\dot{V}O_2$ relationships during normal metabolism (as in Figure 1-11) and during hypermetabolism. During normal, hypometabolic, or hypermetabolic states the normal ratio of delivery to consumption is 5:1. This results in 80% venous saturation (V sat) if the arterial blood is 100% saturated. The isobar for the 5:1 ratio is demonstrated in this diagram, as well as the isobar for the 4:1, 3:1, and 2:1 ratios. Corresponding levels of venous saturation are shown. A state of decreasing oxygen consumption in which consumption is supply dependent occurs when the ratio is less than 2:1. (ⓜ = /min/m²; Sa = arterial saturation.)

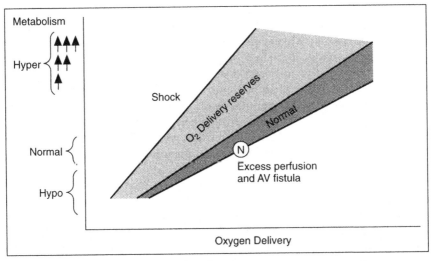

FIGURE 1-13. Interpreting the $\dot{D}O_2/\dot{V}O_2$ diagram. In this diagram the relationships shown in Figures 1-11 and 1-12 are demonstrated without specific numerical values to emphasize the difference between normal relationships, the utilization of oxygen delivery reserves, and shock. (AV = arteriovenous; Ⓝ = normal.)

circumstances the saturation of mixed venous blood (SvO_2) is 80%. (Mixed venous blood must be used for this measurement because the relative extraction by organs served by the superior and inferior vena cava and coronary sinus are quite different.) If an 80% SvO_2 corresponds to a 5:1 ratio, then 75% corresponds to 4:1, 66% to 3:1, 50% to 2:1, and so on. As long as the arterial blood is fully saturated, this holds true regardless of the absolute level of $\dot{D}O_2$ or $\dot{V}O_2$, as shown in Figure 1-12. If the arterial blood is less than fully saturated, the difference between the arterial (SaO_2) and venous saturation corresponds to the oxygen extraction, hence the $\dot{D}O_2/\dot{V}O_2$ ratio. For example, if the arterial blood were 80% saturated and the venous blood were 64% saturated, the ratio would be 5:1.

All of these interrelationships were originally pointed out by Fick in 1870. Fick's axiom is that oxygen consumption via the airway is equal to that in peripheral tissues. His equation for calculating cardiac output is CO = $\dot{V}O_2$ divided by $AV\dot{D}O_2$, which can also be expressed as $AVDO_2$ times the cardiac output equals $\dot{V}O_2$.

In critically ill patients the $\dot{V}O_2$ may be elevated or depressed, but a slight to moderate elevation in the $\dot{V}O_2$ is the most common abnormality in critically ill patients. It will be elevated in proportion to the degree of inflammation (either bacterial or sterile, as in burns and pancreatitis). A febrile patient with pronounced signs of septic toxicity typically has a $\dot{V}O_2$ 1.5 times normal (see Figure 1-8). It is very unusual for a critically ill patient to have a $\dot{V}O_2$ greater than twice the normal value. This occurs only in the setting of severe muscular exercise such as that produced by seizures or tetanus. $\dot{V}O_2$ is decreased in critically ill patients who are hypothermic. In them, just as in normal subjects, a change in $\dot{V}O_2$ is followed promptly by a proportionate change in $\dot{D}O_2$. It is "normal" for a hypermetabolic patient to have a high cardiac output and pulse rate, that is, to be in a "hyperdynamic" state.

Rarely the hyperdynamic response exceeds the increase in $\dot{V}O_2$, as reflected in a ratio higher than 5:1 and as SvO_2 greater than 80%. This can occur when a large arteriovenous fistula is present, either resulting from direct vascular communication or from the hyperperfusion of tissues such as occurs in the setting of portal hypertension with excessive perfusion of the splanchnic viscera. The perfusion of nonmetabolizing tissue such as the reestablishment of flow to a long-ischemic leg or successful cardiac resuscitation after a lengthy cardiac arrest will result in an SvO_2 of more than 90%. Rarely this phenomenon is seen after cellular poisoning, as in the setting of carbon monoxide cytochrome intoxication or end-stage sepsis. An abnormally high SvO_2 also occurs when normal $\dot{D}O_2$ is maintained during hypothermia, such as in the setting of cardiopulmonary bypass during cardiac operations.

Some patients cannot mount an increased $\dot{D}O_2$ in response to an increased $\dot{V}O_2$ because of any combination of hypoxia, anemia, and myocardial failure. If this occurs, the $\dot{D}O_2/\dot{V}O_2$ ratio will be less than 5:1, the $AVDO_2$ widens, the SvO_2 decreases, the amount of oxygen extracted from each deciliter of blood increases, and the patient is using up the systemic oxygen reserves. This

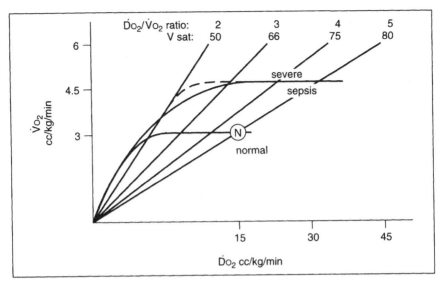

FIGURE 1-14. In the setting of certain conditions such as sepsis and peripheral edema, the biphasic relationship between $\dot{D}O_2/\dot{V}O_2$ becomes blunted and the critical $\dot{D}O_2/\dot{V}O_2$ ratio may be closer to 3:1 than 2:1. The $\dot{D}O_2/\dot{V}O_2$ curve in a normal hypermetabolic condition (exercise) is shown by the dotted line. (Ⓝ = normal.)

increased extraction is perfectly adequate compensation, however, and the patient's condition remains stable as long as the ratio exceeds 2:1. When the various mechanisms of delivery cannot maintain $\dot{D}O_2$ at least twice the $\dot{V}O_2$, supply dependency and ultimately shock occur.

There have been a series of clinical studies allegedly showing that the biphasic relationship is absent and there is a continuous state of $\dot{V}O_2$ supply dependency in patients with the adult respiratory distress syndrome or sepsis. These studies are marred by artifacts of clinical investigation and the results are not supported by the results of laboratory studies in which all the variables can be evaluated. Most investigators agree that a "pathologic oxygen supply dependency" does not exist. However, it appears that the "knee" of the biphasic curve may be shifted to the right in sepsis, making the critical $\dot{D}O_2/\dot{V}O_2$ ratio closer to 3:1 than 2:1 (Figure 1-14). This is probably due to the rate of oxygen diffusion from capillaries to mitochondria in edematous tissues rather than to a specific abnormality in oxidative metabolism.

The shape of the oxyhemoglobin dissociation curve shown in Figure 1-3 changes in the settings of various conditions, moving to the right during acidosis, hypercapnia, and hyperthermia. Although these changes have physiologic importance (for example, facilitating systemic oxygen unloading during ischemia and acidosis), the effects on oxygen content and the relationship to P_{O_2} and saturation are relatively minor compared with the effects of the hemoglobin level on oxygen content.

Implications for Patient Management

For many years Shoemaker has pointed out that patients at risk for multiple-organ failure whose cardiac output, hemoglobin level, and oxygenation are sufficient to maintain normal $\dot{D}O_2/\dot{V}O_2$ ratios (in excess of $4:1$) have less complications and higher survival rates than do patients who cannot maintain normal $\dot{D}O_2$ in relation to their metabolic rates. Similarly, many investigators have shown that patients who cannot mount the response of increased $\dot{D}O_2$ in response to increased metabolism and whose $\dot{D}O_2/\dot{V}O_2$ ratios hover around $2:1$ have lactic acidosis, multiple complications, and a high mortality rate.

Clinical research on $\dot{D}O_2/\dot{V}O_2$ relationships in critically ill patients is notoriously difficult because there are so many variables, many of which cannot be controlled, and because complications and outcome relate to many factors, including the nature of the primary injury or illness in addition to the oxygen kinetic physiologic state. For example, many of the clinical studies performed over the past decade have been conducted in patients whose baseline $\dot{D}O_2/\dot{V}O_2$ ratio was $2:1$ or $3:1$. Individual interventions to raise or lower the $\dot{D}O_2$ in these patients, who were in retrospect on the knee of the $\dot{D}O_2/\dot{V}O_2$ curve, often showed supply dependency. This was interpreted as "pathologic" supply dependency, when in fact the patients were never brought to normal $\dot{D}O_2/\dot{V}O_2$ ratios of $4:1$ or $5:1$. In the laboratory, all the variables can be controlled through the use of complex physiologic preparations. In such studies a normal oxygen kinetic physiologic state was demonstrated in normal animals (Cilley), hypometabolic animals (Sinard), and animals that were in a hypermetabolic state as a result of exercise (Bongiorno) or sepsis (Hirschl).

In critically ill patients therefore, it is a good management policy to maintain $\dot{D}O_2$ greater than four times the $\dot{V}O_2$. If the patient cannot do this through the process of autoregulation, then $\dot{D}O_2$ should be optimized by the transfusion of red blood cells, by improved oxygenation via the lungs, or by an increase in cardiac output brought about by the administration of inotropic drugs. In addition, the ratio can be optimized by decreasing oxygen consumption either by inducing paralysis or by cooling. Several studies have shown that optimizing the $\dot{D}O_2/\dot{V}O_2$ ratio in critically ill patients improves outcome (Tuchschmidt, Yu, Boyd, and Fleming).

Because continuous SvO_2 monitoring is a continuous and direct measurement of the $\dot{D}O_2/\dot{V}O_2$ ratio, it is the ideal way to determine when systemic $\dot{D}O_2$ is optimized and to titrate treatment aimed at optimizing $\dot{D}O_2$ (blood transfusion, FiO_2, PEEP, inotropes) or $\dot{V}O_2$ (cooling). Arterial pulse oximetry and mixed venous saturation monitoring nearly eliminate the need for most of the individual measurements of the components of oxygen delivery (cardiac output and blood gas levels). The ability to monitor these variables continuously using SvO_2 allows interventions to be instituted to maintain normal $\dot{D}O_2/\dot{V}O_2$ relationships before critically low levels are reached.

Monographs and Reviews

Bartlett RH. Post traumatic pulmonary insufficiency. In: Cooper P, Nyhus I, eds. Surgery Annual, 1971. New York: Appleton-Century-Crofts, 1971.
This chapter has concise descriptions of normal and abnormal respiratory physiology in the setting of critical illness. Several figures from this chapter are included in this text.

Bartlett RH. Critical Care. In: Greenfield L, ed. Surgery: scientific principles and practice. Philadelphia: Lippincott, 1992:195–222.
Oxygen kinetics is presented as the background for monitoring and management in critical care.

Bartlett RH. A critical carol: being an essay on anemia, suffocation, starvation, and other forms of intensive care, after the manner of Dickens. Chest 1984;85:687–93.
Written in a most unusual style for scientific journals, this editorial points out some common errors related to oxygen kinetics that occur in critical care management.

Cain SM, Curtis SE. Experimental models of pathologic oxygen supply dependency. Crit Care Med 1991;19:603–12.
For two decades Stephen Cain has been the leading experimental physiologist studying oxygen kinetics. This is an excellent review of experimental studies, focusing on factors that affect oxygen utilization in peripheral tissues.

Dantzker DR, Foresman B, Gutierrez G. Oxygen supply and utilization relationships: a reevaluation. Am Rev Respir Dis 1991;143:675–9.
The authors review previous reports of studies (including their own) that purported to show a pathologic supply dependency, concluding that the $\dot{D}O_2/\dot{V}O_2$ interactions in many cases represent normal physiologic behavior rather than an abnormal manifestation of impaired oxygen extraction.

Edwards JD. Oxygen transport in the critically ill. Intensive Crit Care Dig 1991;10:23–25.
An English intensivist concisely summarizes the literature on oxygen kinetics.

Hirschl RB. Oxygen delivery in the pediatric surgical patient. Curr Sci 1994;6:341–7.
Although written with the pediatric patient in mind, this chapter includes references to most of the modern investigations in clinical oxygen kinetics.

Reinhart K, Eyrich K. Clinical aspects of O_2 transport and tissue oxygenation. Berlin: Springer-Verlag, 1989.
This is the proceedings of a symposium on oxygen transport held in Berlin in 1989. The concepts of simultaneous continuous venous and arterial oximetry are well described.

Russell JA, Phang PT. Oxygen delivery/consumption controversy: approaches to management of critically ill. Am J Respir Crit Care Med 1994;149:533–7.
The Vancouver group has conducted many clinical research studies on oxygen kinetics in critically ill patients, which are summarized in this review. Mathematical coupling in clinical research studies is particularly well described.

White KM. Completing the hemodynamic picture: SvO_2. Heart Lung 1985;14:272–80.
This paper written by critical care nurse Kathleen White is one of the best descriptions of the use of continuous venous saturation monitoring as a guide to oxygen kinetics.

Selected Reports

Bartlett RH, Dechert RE. Oxygen kinetics: pitfalls in clinical research [editorial]. J Crit Care 1990;5:77–80.
The problems and goals in clinical oxygen kinetic research are enumerated.

Boorstein SM, Hirschl RB, Riley MK, Kahan BS, Hultquist KA, Bartlett RH. The effect of norepinephrine infusion on oxygen delivery and consumption in the canine model. J Surg Res 1994;56:251–5.
Norepinephrine increases $\dot{D}O_2$ but also increases $\dot{V}O_2$ in normal dogs. Whenever catecholamines are used to increase cardiac output, a concomitant increase in $\dot{V}O_2$ can be expected based on the primary effects of the drug on systemic metabolism.

Boyd O, Grounds RM, Bennett ED. A randomized clinical trial of the effect of deliberate perioperative increase in oxygen delivery on mortality in high-risk surgical patients. JAMA 1993;270:2699–707.
This prospective randomized controlled study showed that mortality and morbidity were decreased when $\dot{D}O_2$ was optimized in surgical patients.

Cain SM. Oxygen delivery and uptake in dogs during anemic and hypoxic hypoxia. J Appl Physiol 1977;42:228–34.
This landmark report was one of the first to characterize oxygen kinetic relationships in detail.

Cilley RE, Scharenberg AM, Bongiorno PF, Bartlett RH. Low oxygen delivery produced by anemia, hypoxia and low cardiac output. J Surg Res 1991;51:425–33.
All the variables of oxygen transport were carefully controlled in dog experiments.

Clark LC. Monitor and control of blood and tissue oxygen tensions. Trans ASAIO 1956;2:41–48.
The original description of the PO_2 electrode.

DeBacker D, Roman A, Vanderlinden P, et al. The effects of balloon filling into the inferior vena cava on the $\dot{D}O_2/\dot{V}O_2$ relationship. J Crit Care 1992;7:167–73.
$\dot{D}O_2$ was varied in normal and endotoxic dogs by creating transient hypovolemia. Normal oxygen kinetics were demonstrated in both groups.

Fick A. On the measurement of blood quantity in the ventricles of the heart. In: Proceedings of the Physiological, Medical Society of Wurzburg, July 9, 1870.
The original "pencil experiment" describing Fick's axiom and Fick's equation for cardiac output measurement.

Fleming A, Bishop M, Shoemaker W, et al. Prospective trial of supranormal values as goals of resuscitation in severe trauma. Arch Surg 1992;127:1175–81.
This prospective, controlled, randomized study demonstrated better survival and fewer complications when $\dot{D}O_2$ was optimized in trauma patients.

Hirschl RB, Heiss KF, Cilley RE, Hultquist KA, Housner J, Bartlett RH. Oxygen kinetics in experimental sepsis. Surgery 1992;112:37–44.
Septic dogs with peritonitis were found to be hypermetabolic but had normal oxygen kinetic interactions.

Jastremski MS, Chelluri L, Beney KM, Bailly RT. Analysis of the effects of continuous on-line monitoring of mixed venous oxygen saturation on patient outcome and cost effectiveness. Crit Care Med 1989;17:148–152.
When compared with patients monitored using standard pulmonary artery catheters, patients who had mixed venous saturation monitoring catheters

had half as many deleterious hemodynamic events and required half as many cardiac output measurements.

Nelson LD. Continuous venous oximetry in surgical patients. Ann Surg 1986; 203:329–33.
One of the first papers demonstrating the value of venous oximetry in critically ill patients.

Quinn TJ, Weissman C, Kemper M. Continual trending of Fick variables in the critically ill patient. Chest 1991;99:703–7.
These authors have reported on several useful clinical research studies on the monitoring of oxygen kinetics. In this study changes in cardiac output in response to metabolic rate were documented by continuous monitoring.

Ronco JJ, Phang PT, Walley KR, Wiggs B, Fenwick JC, Russel JA. Oxygen consumption is independent of changes in oxygen delivery in severe adult respiratory distress syndrome. Am Rev Respir Dis 1991;143:1267–73.
This paper points out the problems of mathematical coupling when $\dot{V}O_2$ and $\dot{D}O_2$ are calculated from the same primary measurements.

Shoemaker W, Appel PL, Kram HB. Hemodynamic and oxygen transport responses in survivors and nonsurvivors of high-risk surgery. Crit Care Med 1993; 21:977–90.
This is one of many studies conducted by Shoemaker's group demonstrating that critically ill patients who can maintain (or are treated to maintain) optimal $\dot{D}O_2$ have a better outcome.

Sinard JM, Vyas D, Hultquist K, Harb J, Bartlett RH. Effects of moderate hypothermia on oxygen consumption at various oxygen deliveries in a sheep model. J Appl Physiol 1992;72:2428–34.
$\dot{D}O_2$ was controlled by extracorporeal circulation over a wide range during normothermia and hypothermia in sheep.

Swan HJC, Ganz W, Forrester JS, et al. Catheterization of the heart in man with the use of a flow-directed balloon-tipped catheter. N Engl J Med 1970;283:447–51.
The original description of the "Swan-Ganz" catheter.

Tremper KK, Barker SJ. Pulse oximetry. Anesthesiology 1989;70:98–108.
A good description of the principles and applications of arterialized capillary oximetry.

Tuchschmidt J, Fried J, Astiz M, Rackow E. Elevation of cardiac output and oxygen delivery improves outcome in septic shock. Chest 1992;102:216–20.
A prospective, randomized controlled study showed that optimizing $\dot{D}O_2$ resulted in decreased mortality in septic shock patients.

Yu M, Levy MM, Smith P, Takiguchi SA, Miyasaki A, Myers SA. Effect of maximizing oxygen delivery on morbidity and mortality rates in critically ill patients: a prospective, randomized, controlled study. Crit Care Med 1993;21:830–8.
Mortality and morbidity were decreased when $\dot{D}O_2$ was optimized in patients with shock, sepsis, and the adult respiratory distress syndrome. Beneficial effects of optimizing $\dot{D}O_2$ were demonstrated only on subgroup analysis of the entire population.

2

Blood Volume and Hemodynamics

Monitoring and management of systemic perfusion is one of the easier aspects of intensive care. In fact an inordinate amount of attention is paid to blood pressure monitoring and management, sometimes to the exclusion of other more important variables such as oxygen delivery and the metabolic rate. In this section we review cardiac physiology and pathophysiology, cardiac function in relationship to the blood volume and filling pressure, and systemic vascular physiology in the management of hypotension or inadequate systemic perfusion.

Cardiac Function

For purposes of understanding physiology it is useful to think of the functions of the right heart and the left heart as related but independent systems (Figure 2-1). In most circumstances the function of the left heart predominates and the function of the right heart follows passively. This is because the controlling factor that regulates systemic perfusion is the state of contraction or tone in systemic arterioles (commonly referred to as *systemic vascular resistance*). Similarly, cardiac failure in adult patients usually refers to left ventricular failure, and all efforts at monitoring and managing cardiac function are focused on the left ventricular and systemic circulations. The exception to this general rule are those circumstances in which the pulmonary vascular resistance and right ventricular function become the limiting factors in cardiac output. This occurs in the setting of acute or chronic pulmonary hypertension caused by primary pulmonary disease, pulmonary embolism, or right ventricular disease or infarction.

Cardiac function is regulated by a complex set of baroreceptors and chemoreceptors that continually adjust the cardiac rate, the strength of

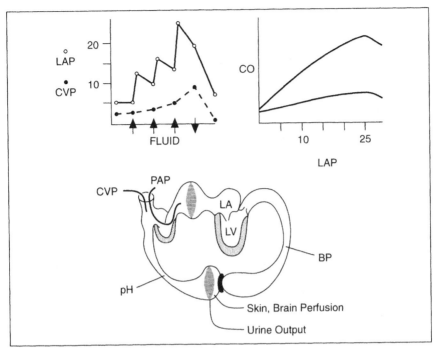

FIGURE 2-1. Right and left heart function related to ventricular filling pressure. (BP = blood pressure; CO = cardiac output; CVP = central venous pressure; LA = left atrium; LV = left ventricle; LAP = left atrial pressure; PAP = pulmonary artery pressure.)

contractility, and the extracellular fluid volume (by diuresis or antidiuresis), all acting to maintain systemic oxygen delivery at four to five times the systemic oxygen consumption. Because normal oxygen consumption is 120 cc/m²/min and the normal arterial oxygen content is 20 cc/dL, normal cardiac output is autoregulated to a level of 3 L/m²/min. If the rate of metabolism increases or decreases, neural and humoral reflexes come into play to readjust the cardiac output proportionately. If the arterial blood oxygen content decreases because of anemia or hypoxemia, cardiac output increases until normal system oxygen delivery is reestablished (see Figure 1-6). If cardiac output decreases because of hypovolemia, catecholamine secretion increases and this results in an increased cardiac rate and contractility to maintain normal systemic oxygen delivery until transcapillary refilling or exogenous treatment causes the blood volume to return to normal. Any or all of these complex interactions may be going on at the same time in a critically ill patient. To assess these factors in the critically ill patient, we estimate cardiac output, blood volume, and filling pressure based on physical examination findings. Specifically we examine the quality and numerical values of

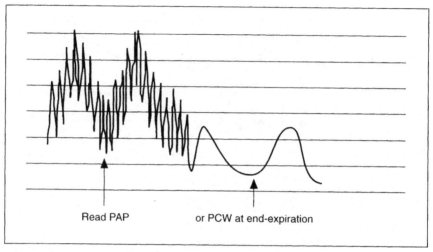

FIGURE 2-2. Pulmonary artery pressure tracing (PAP) in a patient on a mechanical ventilator. Pressures are read at end-expiration (functional residual capacity). The pulmonary capillary wedged pressure (PCW) is measured when the inflow is occluded with a balloon upstream from the tip of the catheter.

the pulse pressure, the adequacy of urine output and brain function, the warmth and perfusion of the skin, and the endogenous autoregulation required to maintain perfusion (tachycardia and chest wall cardiac impulse). All of these findings give us a reasonable estimate of cardiac output. Examination of the lungs for signs of vascular congestion and examination of the visible veins in the neck to estimate venous pressure gives us some determination of the filling pressure. Often these physical findings are adequate to establish a diagnosis and allow management to be instituted. If this level of monitoring is not satisfactory to solve the clinical problems, direct measurement of the filling pressure of the right heart (central venous pressure) or the left heart (pulmonary artery pressure) is required (Figure 2-2). Placement of a pulmonary artery catheter allows us to measure cardiac output by thermodilution and, more importantly, to sample mixed venous blood for the purpose of saturation measurements, which yields the ratio of systemic oxygen delivery to oxygen consumption. All intrathoracic pressures are measured at the end of expiration (functional residual capacity [FRC]). This may be only a single heartbeat (Figure 2-2).

From all these measurements we can determine whether cardiac output is normal for the filling pressure of the left ventricle or whether contractility is decreased. In the latter case cardiac output will be lower than that predicted for a given filling pressure. These relationships are described in the familiar Frank-Starling curve, which is shown in Figure 2-3. If the measurements are in the normal range, then myocardial function can be assumed to be normal. If the measurements are to the right of the normal range, then cardiac

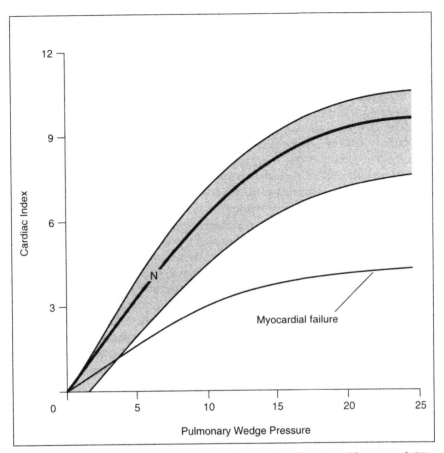

FIGURE 2-3. Frank-Starling curve describing cardiac function. The normal (N) relationships are in the shaded area.

function itself is compromised as the result of valvular disease, extrinsic pressure such as pericardial tamponade, or, most commonly, a decrease in contractility.

Cardiac Function, Blood Volume, and Filling Pressure

The filling pressure already described and identified in Figure 2-3 reflects the relationship between cardiac function and the effective blood volume. If cardiac function and anatomy are normal, then blood volume, filling pressure, and cardiac function are related, as shown in the normal area of the Frank-Starling curve. The intake and output of fluid and salt are autoregulated to maintain the filling pressure of the left ventricle at approximately 10 mm Hg. Under normal circumstances it is almost impossible for a healthy person to become hypervolemic. The ingestion of water, even in huge amounts, has minimal effect on blood volume because the water is distributed throughout the total body water, only a very small fraction of which is in the blood volume. Moreover, diuresis occurs promptly, maintaining the total body water content normal or close to it. The voluntary ingestion of very large amounts of salt and water could result in hypervolemia, but this fluid would be distributed throughout the entire extracellular space, only a fourth of which would be in the plasma volume. In this circumstance, diuresis would occur more slowly, responding to volume receptors rather than to osmoreceptors. In fact, the extracellular space can be overloaded for days or weeks with a minimal autogenous diuretic response. However, extracellular fluid expansion (generalized edema) is usually associated with a normal blood volume. It is important to remember this fact when dealing with a critically ill patient who has fluid overload. Gross expansion of the extracellular space with all the deleterious effects of tissue edema can and often does exist in concert with a perfectly normal blood volume. In other words, a pulmonary capillary wedge pressure of 5 to 10 mm Hg does not rule out the presence of fluid overload as the cause of pulmonary or gastrointestinal tract dysfunction, for example. If hypervolemia does occur because of gross expansion of the extracellular space or because of the intravenous infusion of fluids or blood, the result will be an increase in left atrial pressure (reflected in the pulmonary artery pressure), central venous pressure, and arterial pulse pressure. These changes are shown in Figure 2-4.

Like hypervolemia, hypovolemia rarely occurs in the normal person. However, short periods of voluntary starvation or short periods of acute disease such as diarrhea or vomiting can result in hypovolemia rather quickly. The fluid losses in these circumstances are extracellular losses, which are relatively slowly reflected as changes in the blood volume. However, even a minor decrease in the extracellular fluid volume leads to antidiuresis as soon as hypovolemia is reflected by decreased arterial filling pressures (see Figure 2-4). Autoregulatory mechanisms cause cardiac output to increase to compensate for this. In the event of bleeding, the change in blood volume is immediate and is immediately reflected in the operation of these compensatory mechanisms. If the bleeding stops before a critical level of exsanguination is reached, the normal combination of hydrostatic and osmotic forces that control the flow of salt and water at the capillary level results in the net transfer of extracellular fluid back into the plasma volume (so-called transcapillary refilling), which restores normal blood volume, albeit with hemodilution.

In critically ill patients, our concern about the possible development of hypotension and ineffective perfusion, although it may be appropriate, usually results in the intravenous infusion of salt and water in quantities that exceed losses. Consequently, most patients in the intensive care unit (ICU) have edema (worse in areas of injury or inflammation), anemia, dilutional hypoproteinemia, and a compensatory increase in cardiac output. These

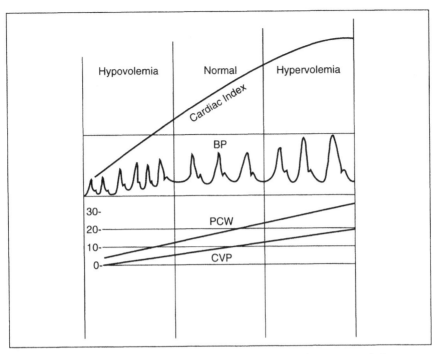

FIGURE 2-4. The effects of changes in blood volume when myocardial function is normal. Hypervolemia results in an increased filling pressures and expanded arterial pulse pressure. Hypovolemia results in a decreased filling pressure and narrowed pulse pressure. (BP = blood pressure; CVP = central venous pressure; PCW = pulmonary capillary wedge pressure.)

patients are tachycardiac in response to anemia, even though their blood volume and filling pressures are normal and their total body extracellular fluid content is excessive. All of these factors are reflected in the autoregulatory mechanisms designed to maintain systemic oxygen delivery at four to five times the consumption level. If arterial saturation is close to 100%, then cardiac function is "normal" for that patient if the venous saturation is in the range of 75% to 80%.

Measuring Blood Volume

Blood volume can be measured by the dilution of specific indicators such as tagged albumin or tagged red blood cells. However, from a practical point of view, blood volume is no longer measured in critically ill patients because its exact measurement is only important as it relates to cardiac function, and this relationship can be determined form the Frank-Starling curve shown in Figure 2-3.

Definitions and formulas related to hemodynamics are given in Table 2-1.

TABLE 2-1. Hemodynamics

Abbreviation	Definition	Formula	Normal value
CO	Cardiac output	—	3.2 L/min/m^2
CI	Cardiac index	CO/m^2	3.2 L/min/m^2
PAP	Pulmonary artery pressure	—	25/10 mm Hg
PCW	Pulmonary capillary wedge pressure	—	5–10 mm Hg
RAP (CVP)	Right arterial pressure (central venous pressure)	—	2–5 mm Hg
BP	Systemic artery pressure	—	120/80 mm Hg
SV	Stroke volume	CO ÷ rate	
SI*	Stroke index	CI ÷ rate	45 mL/beat
SVRI*	Systemic vascular resistance index	$\frac{MAP - RAP}{CI}$	25–30 units
PVRI*	Pulmonary vascular resistance index	$\frac{MPAP - LAP}{CI}$	1–2 units
LVSWI*	Left ventricular stroke work index	SI × MAP × 0.0144	50 gm·m^{-1}·m^2
RVSWI*	Right ventricular stroke work index	SI × MPAP × 0.0144	10 gm·m^{-1}·m^2
RPP	Rate pressure product	BP × rate	12,000
Fick equation		$CO = \frac{\dot{V}O_2}{AVDO_2}$	

*Use CI to calculate derived variables.
AVDO$_2$ = arteriovenous oxygen content difference; LAP = left atrial pressure; MAP = mean arterial pressure; MPAP = mean pulmonary artery pressure; RAP = right atrial pressure; $\dot{V}O_2$ = oxygen consumption per minute.

Measurement of Vascular Pressures

The measurement of arterial blood pressure by auscultation and balloon cuff occlusion is a common practice, but subject to many errors of measurement and interpretation. In most critically ill patients, arterial blood pressure is measured directly through a catheter inserted into a systemic artery. Direct measurement of the arterial blood pressure by means of a transducer and electrical display or recording device is also subject to errors in measurement and interpretation, but it is much more accurate than conventional sphygmomanometry. Assuming that the intra-arterial measurement system is working correctly, direct arterial blood pressure measurements are the gold standard in the ICU. It is never necessary, in fact it is usually misleading, to "check" the direct measurement against the "cuff" measurements. Originally arterial blood pressure was measured directly in the aorta through catheters placed via the femoral artery. Now the radial artery at the wrist is most commonly used for continuous blood pressure measurement because it is easily accessible and the complication rate associated with this method is very low. Right atrial or central venous pressure is measured by a catheter that has been advanced into the area of the right atrium and attached to a manometer or a transducer. Pulmonary artery pressure is similarly measured by a catheter that has been placed in a lobar or segmental pulmonary artery. The sequential pressure changes observed in the right atrium, right ventricle, pulmonary artery, and wedged positions are used to guide the catheter into this position. The position is verified by a chest x-ray.

Pressures throughout the cardiovascular system reflect the contractility of the upstream ventricle, the downstream arterial resistance, and to a small extent the viscosity of the blood. In addition, the vascular pressures are affected by respiration. The effects of respiration on arterial pressure are minimal and usually ignored, but its effects on intrathoracic pressures are very important. By general agreement, intrathoracic intravascular pressures are measured at FRC, that is, at the end of an exhaled breath (see Figure 2-2). If both the heart rate and respiratory rate are rapid, this point of measurement may be only a single heartbeat. For this reason it is necessary to obtain the right atrial pressure, pulmonary artery pressure, and pulmonary capillary wedge pressure from a storage oscilloscope or paper tracing rather than from a digital output, which tends to average the pressure over many heartbeats and many respiratory cycles. The wedged pressure was originally described by Dexter and is the pressure obtained when an end-hole catheter is advanced into the pulmonary vasculature until it is wedged in a small artery. The pressure obtained at the tip of the catheter is a measure of the pressure in the pulmonary capillaries, which in turn is a measure of the pressure in the left atrium and the left ventricle at end-diastole (if the mitral valve is normal). Right heart catheterization moved from the cardiac catheterization laboratory to the patient's bedside in the ICU when Edwards Laboratories developed a long, thin catheter with a small balloon near the tip. Inflation of the balloon (usually) carries the catheter along with the flowing blood through the right heart chambers into the pulmonary artery, thus eliminating the need for fluoroscopy. Edwards' original catheter was tested and described by Los Angeles cardiologists Swan and Ganz and as a result became known as the *Swan-Ganz catheter*. This device has been so useful and so widely recognized that it has joined our lexicon of noun-verbs. We often hear that a patient is going to be "swaned" or that the Swan readings are such-and-such. Pulmonary artery catheters have undergone many modifications since the original device came into use and it is grammatically and historically more correct to speak of *pulmonary artery catheters* and Frank-Starling measurements. However, we don't object too much, recognizing the importance of acknowledging our heritage.

If the intrathoracic pressure at FRC is higher than the atmospheric pressure, this condition is referred to as *positive end-expiratory pressure* (PEEP). PEEP is commonly used in the treatment of critically ill patients in an attempt to maintain inflation of the alveoli served by small airways that collapse at lower pressures. PEEP levels as high as 25 cm H_2O are sometimes used. To measure intravascular pressures when PEEP is used, it is best to ignore the PEEP and measure and report the pressure regardless of the level of PEEP. The reason for this is that the end-expiratory pressure measured at the airway is different from, and higher than, the pressure measured at the tip of intravascular catheters because the chest is not a closed box but rather an expansile box with a very floppy bottom (the diaphragm).

In addition to the effects of respiration and expiratory pressure, the position of the patient affects the resulting measurement of the intravascular pressures because of the simple weight of blood when the catheter tip is in a dependent position. Movement of the patient may also change the relationship between the tip of the catheter and the electronic transducer. These problems are solved by placing the manometer or transducer at the level of the left atrium when making measurements. This can and should be done when the patient is in a lateral position, sitting up, or prone. It is not necessary to put the patient in a supine position to measure the hemodynamic pressures.

Measurement of Cardiac Output

Although there are many ways to measure the output of the heart, only two are generally used in the ICU: the indicator dilution method using a cold solution as the indicator and the Fick method. In the indicator dilution method a small bolus of a measurable indicator (originally Evans blue or indocyanine green dye) is injected rapidly into the central venous system (the exact location is not important). The concentration of the indicator is measured continuously downstream, either in the pulmonary artery or in a systemic artery. The ventricle acts as a mixing chamber that distributes the bolus of injectate into the ventricular volume, typically about 100 mL (Figure 2-5). If the cardiac output is high, the volume of dyed blood will move through the circulation very quickly, so that the concentration at the point of measurement rises quickly to a high peak value then disappears quickly. (The tail of the disappearance curve will be distorted by some of the dye that has already gone through the entire systemic circulation and recirculated back to the point of measurement.) If the cardiac output is very low, the volume of dyed blood moves relatively slowly and the concentration rises slowly at the point of measurement, then slowly declines as the indicator is washed through. The area under the curve describing the concentration of the indicator is a measure of the total volume of blood into which the indicator has been dispersed, from the point of injection to the point of measurement. This is known as the *central blood volume*. The exact quantity can be calculated by knowing the exact quantity of indicator injected and the extent to which it has been diluted. Similarly the time that it takes half the central blood volume to go past the point of measurement can be measured and described as the mean transit time. Therefore, if we know the volume of blood and the time of passage, we can calculate the volume of blood that would flow through the ventricle, or ventricles, per minute, which is in fact the cardiac output. At one time, part of this measurement was done by

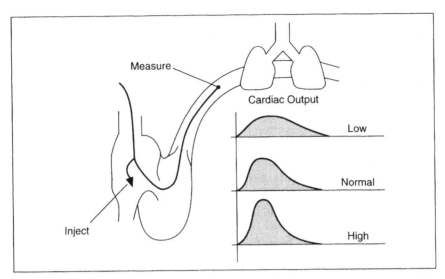

FIGURE 2-5. Indicator dilution cardiac output (C.O.) measurement using cold solution as the indicator. A bolus of cold crystalloid solution is injected into the central venous circulation (any central venous catheter will do), and temperature is measured near the tip of the catheter in the pulmonary artery. Typical thermal dilution curves are shown.

cutting out the paper tracing of the dye concentration and balancing it on a straight edge to determine the time when half the indicator had passed the measurement point or to determine the dye concentration halfway between maximal and minimal. This method was reduced to a series of formulas by Stewart and Hamilton, who are credited with popularizing the indicator dilution method. The indicator dilution method involving central venous injection and systemic arterial sampling was used in ICUs for many years but was cumbersome because of dye gradually accumulated in the patient, requiring frequent recalibration that involved diluting a sample of the injectate with aliquots of blood. This problem was eliminated when it was discovered that temperature could be used as the indicator, and this consisted in the injection of a small bolus of room temperature or, better yet, iced crystalloid solution. Moreover, by including a sensitive thermistor on the tip of a pulmonary artery catheter, the thermal indicator dilution method could be used easily and repeatedly in any patient with a pulmonary artery catheter in place. Thus the thermal dilution method of determining cardiac output has been widely used in ICUs for the past twenty years.

Like any dye dilution method, thermal dilution cardiac outputs are subject to many methodologic artifacts. The colder the solution, the more detectable the differences, but iced fluid changes temperature when going through conduit tubing and a warm intravascular segment of catheter. The most accurate results are obtained when the injectate bolus is injected very quickly, but incorporating the injection lumen into the wall of the pulmonary artery catheter necessarily made that lumen very small, such that rapid (half-second) injection is not possible. The timing of the injection in relation to the respiratory cycle affects the reproducibility of the measurement. Because of these artifacts, the usual practice is to obtain three or four indicator dilution curves, discard the curves that show irregularities, and average the results of the remaining curves. The net result of all this is that thermal dilution cardiac outputs are accurate $\pm 10\%$ under the very best of circumstances. Nonetheless, it is certainly worthwhile to know if the cardiac index is 2, 4, or 6 L/min. It is important to remember, however, that in all calculations based on cardiac output, the errors in measurement will simply be magnified. The principles of thermal dilution cardiac output are depicted in Figure 2-5.

The gold standard method of measuring cardiac output is the one described by Adolph Fick. Fick never actually measured cardiac output but simply postulated that it could be done if there were a way to measure the mixed venous and arterial oxygen content and oxygen consumption at the airway. By measuring the oxygen consumption per minute, and by knowing the arteriovenous oxygen concentration difference ($AVDO_2$) in cubic centimeters of oxygen per deciliter of blood, it is simple arithmetic to determine how many deciliters of blood pass through the lung in a minute. The Fick method works well regardless of the status of lung function because of the Fick axiom, which assumes that the amount of oxygen absorbed across the lung is exactly equal to the amount of oxygen utilized in peripheral tissues. Perhaps a better way to describe the Fick equation would be to divide the $AVDO_2$ into the amount of oxygen consumed in the process of metabolism in peripheral tissues. Measuring cardiac output using the Fick technique requires getting a sample of mixed venous blood (hence necessitating use of a pulmonary artery catheter) and a sample of arterial blood (hence the need for an arterial catheter) as well as accurate measurement of oxygen consumption at the airway. The error in each of these measurements is a few percent, so that even the Fick cardiac output method has an overall error rate of $\pm 5\%$. The principles involved in measuring cardiac output using the Fick method are depicted in Figure 2-6.

More accurate, simpler, or, best of all, continuous methods of cardiac output measurement would be desirable in the management of critically ill patients. Some of the other methods that have been utilized include indicator dilution using radioisotopes with external counting; ultrasonic measurement of the velocity of flow through large vessels or cardiac chambers, with calculations based on the measured or estimated cross-sectional area of the vessel; transthoracic electrical impedance measurement analysis of the arterial pulse waveform; and continuous thermal dilution using slow infusions or heated wires to produce a temperature gradient. To date none of these methods has proved reliable enough to replace the bolus thermal indicator dilution method.

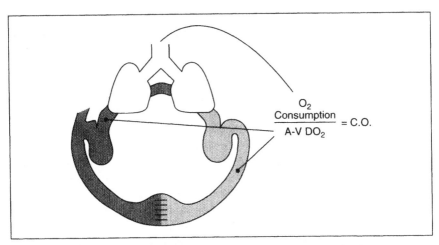

FIGURE 2-6. Cardiac output (C.O.) measured by the Fick method requires measurement of the oxygen content in arterial and venous blood and the oxygen consumption at the airway. (A-V DO$_2$ = arteriovenous oxygen content difference.)

Systemic and Regional Blood Flow

All of this discussion has regarded cardiac output as if blood flow were ideally distributed to each of the various organ systems. In fact, this is not usually the case. Even in periods of high and low cardiac outputs, the organs that need increased oxygen delivery (that is, blood flow) get the extra blood flow at the expense of other organs that need it less. This autoregulation is based primarily on the maintenance of total systemic vascular resistance, as determined by the arteriolar tone in all organs throughout the vascular system. In some organs, such as the heart and brain, constant blood flow is maintained over a wide range of inflow pressures. In other organs, such as the kidney, blood flow is more sensitive to the arterial pressure, or more accurately, arteriolar resistance regulates organ blood flow in a fairly active fashion. The management of regional or organ-specific blood flow is rarely possible or even considered in the management of the critically ill patient. Notable exceptions are the administration of vasopressin and glucagon to selectively increase or decrease splanchnic blood flow and the induction of hypocapnic alkalosis to decrease cerebral blood flow. Low doses of dopamine are said to selectively improve renal blood flow, although this phenomenon may primarily be the result of a generalized increase in cardiac output.

In the context of peripheral circulation, a word should be said about vascular resistance. The calculation of "resistance" is a useful shorthand means of describing the interrelationships of cardiac output and systemic or pulmonary blood pressure, but it is no more than that. It is impossible to measure resistance. Resistance is simply a calculation in which blood pressure is divided by blood flow. The results should be expressed as Wood units, or millimeters of mercury per liter per minute per square meter. It is naive to apply other laws of fluid dynamic physics, which are described for the flow of newtonian fluids through rigid tubes, and it is ridiculous to convert resistance units to dyne $\cdot$ s^{-1} $\cdot$ cm^{-5} as if the resulting number will somehow be more accurate. (Multiplying Wood units times 79.9 to express resistance is a common practice but has no rational basis.) All cardiovascular measurements should be normalized to body weight or body surface area, and this is particularly true of resistance calculations. Cardiac index rather than cardiac output should always be used for resistance calculations to compare the individual patient's values with the theoretically normal values. For example, both a 4-year-old child with a blood pressure of 90/60 mm Hg and a well-trained 300-pound (135-kg) adult athlete with a blood pressure of 110/80 mm Hg have a normal cardiac index. The calculated systemic vascular resistance based on the cardiac index is the same for both and is normal. If the calculated systemic vascular resistance were based on cardiac output, it would be "pathologically" high in the child and "pathologically" low in the athlete.

Management of Hypotension and Hypoperfusion

Our algorithm for hemodynamic management is shown in Figure 2-7. Despite all of the foregoing discussion, the first sign that brings hemodynamic problems to light is often low blood pressure. If we identify a patient who has low blood pressure (or tachycardia, confusion, syncope, or narrow pulse pressure) as one whose systemic oxygen delivery may be inadequate to meet metabolic needs (that is, shock), our first response is to assess venous pressure by physical examination. If the venous pressure is high, we presume the problem is related to the heart or some mechanical obstruction to blood flow. If the venous pressure is low, we presume the problem is attributable to hypovolemia or systemic vasodilatation. If the patient does not respond to initial simple management, more detailed monitoring is necessary in the form of a central venous pressure catheter. If simple monitoring yields a diagnosis, we can proceed to implement appropriate treatment. If signs of inadequate blood flow based on venous pressure measurements persist despite treatment, then transfer of the patient to the ICU and direct monitoring of pulmonary artery pressure, saturation, and cardiac output are necessary.

With a pulmonary artery catheter in place we can determine whether oxygen delivery is adequate to meet metabolic needs (venous saturation is greater than 65% assuming that arterial saturation is more than 95%). If this is so, then no further acute treatment is needed. If this is not so, then an appropriate blood volume expander should be given until the wedge pressure exceeds 10 mm Hg. The appropriate blood volume expander may be blood, crystalloid solution, or plasma substitute, depending on the presumed or proven fluid loss that led to the hypovolemia.

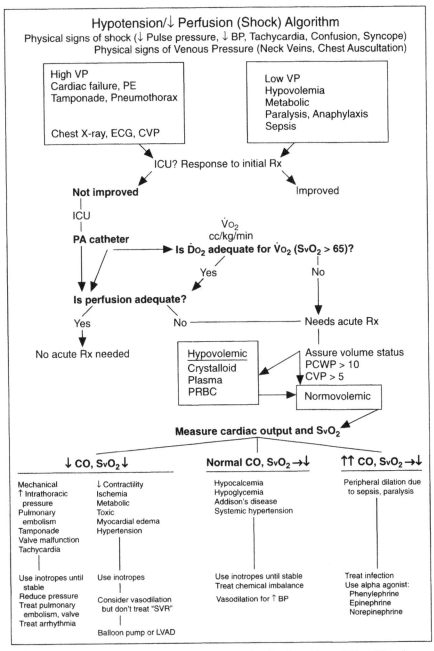

FIGURE 2-7. Hemodynamic management (shock) algorithm. (BP = blood pressure; CO = cardiac output; CVP = central venous pressure; $\dot{D}o_2$ = oxygen delivery; ECG = electrocardiogram; LVAD = left ventricular assist device; P = pressure; PA = pulmonary artery; PCWP = pulmonary capillary wedge pressure; PE = pulmonary embolism; PRBC = packed red blood cells; SVR = systemic vascular resistance; VP = venous pressure; SvO_2 = venous saturation.)

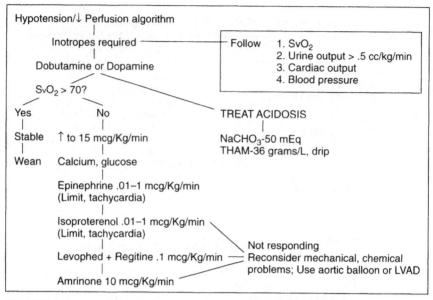

FIGURE 2-8. Inotrope algorithm. (LVAD = left ventricular assist device; SvO_2 = venous saturation.)

If despite adequate filling pressure cardiac output is still decreased, and/or venous saturation is less than 65%, then the cause is probably related to cardiac function and appropriate treatment can be undertaken. If mechanical factors are ruled out and contractility is the limiting factor, then inotropic drugs are the appropriate treatment (Figure 2-8 and Table 2-2). If cardiac output is high and hypotension persists, the cause may be systemic vasodilatation (resulting from sepsis, paralysis, or vasodilating drugs) or the problem may be metabolic in origin (hypoglycemia, hypocalcemia, or Addison's disease). If blood pressure is normal or high and cardiac output is decreased despite adequate filling pressures, then the problem may be systemic hypertension with or without decreased contractility. Only in the latter circumstance is it appropriate to administer systemic vasodilating drugs (Figure 2-9).

If the patient is already systemically vasodilated as the result of the primary disease, the cardiac output will be high and the blood pressure (therefore the calculated resistance) will be low. This occurs with the loss of vasomotor tone stemming from anaphylaxis or acute spinal cord injury but is most commonly due to systemic sepsis. The lipopolysaccharide endotoxin elaborated by most gram-negative bacteria is the most common cause of the septic shock syndrome, although it can also be associated with gram-positive and even yeast infection. Some of the vasodilatation is undoubtedly due to the activation of neutrophils and macrophages, with the attendant systemic production of interleukins, leukotrienes, and platelet-derived cytokines. However, the major mechanisms responsible for this is mediated by tumor

TABLE 2-2. "Pressor" Drugs

Drug	Contractility (Inotropic)	SA Node Rate (Chronotropic)	Vasoconstriction	Vasodilatation	Renal Perfusion	Cardiac Output	Systemic Vascular Resistance	Blood Pressure	$\dot{V}O_2$, $\dot{V}CO_2$, REE
Isoproterenol	+++	+++	0	+++	↑ or ↓	↑	↓	↓ to ↑	↑
Dobutamine	+++	0 to +	0 to +	0 to +	↑	↑	↓	0 to ↑	↑
Dopamine	+++	+	0 to +++	0	↑ or ↓	↑	↓ or ↑	0 to ↑	↑
Epinephrine	+++	+++	+++	++	↓	↑	↓	↑	↑
Norepinephrine	++	++	+++	0	↓	↓ or ↑	↑	↑	↑
Ephedrine	++	++	+	0 to +	↓	↑	↓ or ↑	↑	↑
Phenylephrine	0	0	+++	0	↓	↓	↑	↑	↑

REE = resting energy expenditure; SA = sinoatrial; $\dot{V}O_2$ = oxygen consumption; $\dot{V}CO_2$ = CO_2 production.
+ = minor; ++ = moderate; +++ = major; ↑ = increased; ↓ = decreased.

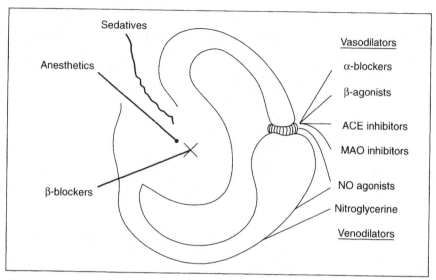

FIGURE 2-9. Drugs used to treat acute hypertension. (ACE = angiotensin-converting enzyme; MAO = monoamine oxidase; NO = nitric oxide.)

necrosis factor, which is elaborated by macrophages. This factor causes vasodilation by activating the production of nitric oxide at the arteriolar level. Because vascular resistance is one of the major controllers of cardiac output, when vascular resistance decreases, cardiac output increases, thus the patient with severe systemic sepsis is most likely to be febrile, tachycardic, hypotensive, alert and awake despite the hypotension, and oliguric with a very high cardiac output; therefore the calculated resistance will be low. The patient's condition is described as "hyperdynamic," but this is a helpful normal response to systemic infection. It is more worrisome if the patient with sepsis does not have a hyperdynamic response. The hyperdynamic state associated with sepsis or anaphylaxis is similar to the hyperdynamic state associated with extensive exercise. One major difference is that in sepsis the capacitance veins, as well as the arteriolar constrictors, are dilated, capillary permeability is often increased, and relative hypovolemia complicates the picture. Because of this, a severely septic patient may initially exhibit hypotension and a normal or low cardiac output, only to progress to the classic hyperdynamic state once adequate volume resuscitation has been achieved.

Hemodynamic treatment of the hyperdynamic state associated with sepsis is somewhat controversial, but rather obvious lessons can be drawn from the treatment of anaphylaxis. The brain, heart, and kidney are organs that can autoregulate blood flow but need a certain mean pressure to maintain adequate perfusion. The first goal then is to restore some level of systemic arteriolar tone using alpha-agonists such as phenylephrine or epinephrine. Remember that these catecholamines increase oxygen consumption as well as vascular tone and heart rate. The final result could be a decrease in the

TABLE 2-3. Hemodynamic Axioms

1. PCWP reflects the left ventricular filling pressure (LAP), which depends **only** on blood volume and myocardial muscle status. LAP = LVEDP if mitral valve is normal.
2. PCWP **does not** reflect extracellular fluid volume; PCWP is generally **not** related to overhydration.
3. PCWP is equal to the pulmonary artery diastolic pressure if the heart rate is < 90 beats/min.
4. RAP (CVP) is always lower than PCWP, except when pulmonary vascular resistance is grossly elevated.
5. Resistance is just a calculation, not a measurement. The units are pressure per flow or millimeters of mercury per liter per minute per meter^2 (usually referred to as *Wood units*). If you multiply Wood units times 79.9, you can express resistance as dyne $\cdot$ s^{-1} $\cdot$ cm^{-5}, but why bother?
6. Use **mean** pressure and cardiac **index** to calculate derived variables (resistance, stroke index, stroke work index).
7. An elevated systemic vascular resistance index is almost always caused by low cardiac output, rarely by primary vasospasm. Treat the cardiac output not the "resistance."

CVP = central venous pressure; LAP = left atrial pressure; LVEDP = left ventricular end-diastolic pressure; PCWP = pulmonary capillary wedge pressure; RAP = right atrial pressure.

---

ratio of systemic oxygen delivery to oxygen consumption. The use of a drug such as dopamine or isoproterenol that has primarily inotropic effects to improve cardiac output is not a good first choice. Turning off the entire hyperdynamic response with beta-blockers, for example, decreases the pulse rate and cardiac output, and therefore appears to increase the calculated resistance but actually increases mortality in the setting of septic inflammatory shock. Of course the most important step in the care of patients with sepsis is to find and treat the primary source of infection.

In summary, the principles involved in hemodynamic monitoring and management are simple: make accurate measurements, rely on primary data rather than on calculated variables whenever possible, understand the differences between blood volume and extracellular volume, and use the measurements to select appropriate drugs and titrate effective blood levels. Some of these principles are summarized in the list of hemodynamic axioms in Table 2-3.

Electrocardiography

The body surface measurement of the electrical potential generated by the conduction system of the heart has not changed a great deal since the time of Einthoven and Wilson. The concept of continuous cardiographic monitoring was introduced by Lown and Levine 40 years ago and remains the mainstay of treatment in coronary care units. In any general ICU almost every possible arrhythmia is seen and treated almost every day. There are dozens of excellent books, not the least of which is the standard *Advanced Cardiac Life*

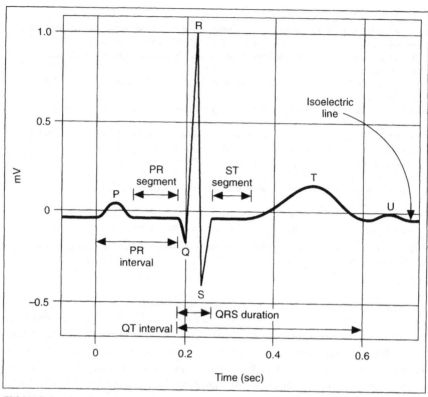

FIGURE 2-10. Elements of the normal electrocardiogram seen in lead II.

Support Manual, and it is not necessary or appropriate to review electrocardiography and arrhythmia management here. The simple practical approach that follows is adequate for recognizing and managing 99% of the cardiac rhythm problems encountered in the ICU. The details of the normal electrocardiogram are reviewed in Figure 2-10. Although the sweep speed and the gain on monitoring oscilloscopes are variable and adjustable, physicians and nurses who spend time in ICUs get quite good at recognizing even esoteric arrhythmias from a glance at the oscilloscope tracing. However, to interpret the fine details such as intervals and voltage, it is necessary to make a paper printout of the tracing with a properly calibrated and timed electrocardiograph machine. When this is done, such elements as the PR interval, the PR segment, and the ST segment can be identified, quantitated, and compared. These intervals are usually measured in lead II, although the placement of electrodes in patients in the ICU can be quite variable. Before any significant diagnosis is made or treatment is undertaken on the basis of the electrocardiographic findings, it is wise to obtain a standard 12-lead electrocardiogram to evaluate the electrical conduction of the heart from all directions. Some of the common drugs and conditions that affect conduction are summarized in Table 2-4.

TABLE 2-4. Drugs and Conditions that Affect the Myocardial Conduction System

Electrocardiographic Feature	Normal	Increased	Decreased
PR interval	1.2–2	AV block	Nodal disease, WPW syndrome
QT interval	0.3–0.4	Low calcium and magnesium levels; lidocaine; quinidine; MI	High calcium, potassium, and magnesium levels; digitalis
T wave	0.25 mV	Raised potassium level; ischemia	—

AV = atrioventricular; MI = myocardial infarction; WPW = Wolff-Parkinson-White syndrome.

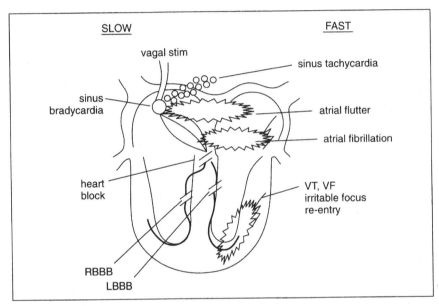

FIGURE 2-11. The common causes of cardiac arrhythmia. (LBBB = left bundle-branch block; RBBB = right bundle-branch block; stim = stimulation; VF = ventricular fibrillation; VT = ventricular tachycardia.)

Arrhythmias

At the risk of insulting my colleagues who devote their entire career to the study and treatment of disturbances of the cardiac rhythm, all of the arrhythmias that affect patients in the ICU can be classified as too fast or too slow, atrial or ventricular, and hemodynamically important or unimportant. The slow arrhythmias are the result of vagal stimulation, sinus node abnormalities, hypercalcemia or hypermagnesemia, or heart block. The common fast arrhythmias are caused by the spontaneous or accelerated firing of parts of the conduction system produced by catechol drugs and hormones, hypokalemia, digitalis, and electrical irritability (Figure 2-11). These arrhythmias may originate at the atrial level, in the conduction system itself, or at the ventricular level. A list of the common causes of arrhythmias, classified in this fashion, is presented in Table 2-5.

The treatment of arrhythmias in patients in the ICU always brings to mind the scene from *Raiders of the Lost Ark* in which a villain with a large sword is threatening to kill the hero, Indiana Jones, who has only a small whip. After parrying thrusts of the sword and sidestepping ever-closer slashes, Indiana Jones becomes bored with the encounter, pulls out a gun, and shoots the villain. We have a long list of drugs that can be used quite successfully to treat all manner of arrhythmias, but if the drugs fail or are not working fast enough, we simply pull out our DC fibrillator (another Bernard Lown invention) or our handy pacemaker and use it to solve the problem. We almost always win. The algorithm for choosing drugs or electricity is shown in Figure 2-12.

Most of the bradyarrhythmias that arise in patients in the ICU are caused by vagal stimulation. Most mysterious intermittent bradyarrhythmias are the result of such mechanical problems as an endotracheal tube or tracheostomy tube positioned near the carina, a nasogastric tube lying in a particularly irritable area of the nasal pharynx, sutures holding chest tubes that pull on the chest wall when the patient moves, or a too full stomach or urinary bladder. These simple assessments and the use of old-fashioned atropine are sometimes forgotten, and they are easier solutions than the insertion of a transvenous pacemaker. Even patients with complete heart block can be managed very successfully with isoproterenol or epinephrine until pacing wires can be electively placed.

Unlike bradyarrhythmias, sometimes the best first solution to tachyarrhythmias is the defibrillator. Lidocaine often eliminates the problem of frequent premature ventricular contractions, and adenosine or verapamil will usually control supraventricular tachycardias, but like Indiana Jones in *Raiders of the Lost Ark*, we have our big gun handy and we are justifiably quick to use it if pharmacologic interventions are not successful.

TABLE 2-5. Common Causes of Arrhythmias by Site of Origin

Site	Slow	Fast
Atrial	Vagal stimulus, sinus bradycardia, sick sinus, medications	Catecholamines, medications, sinus tachycardia, atrial flutter, atrial fibrillation
Conduction	Wandering pacemaker; first-, second-, and third-degree heart block; PACs	Wenckebach's disease, Torsades de pointes, PVCs
Ventricular	Standstill, diastolic arrest, potassium	Ventricular tachycardia, ventricular fibrillation, catecholamines

PACs = premature atrial contractions; PVCs = premature ventricular contractions.

2. Blood Volume and Hemodynamics   45

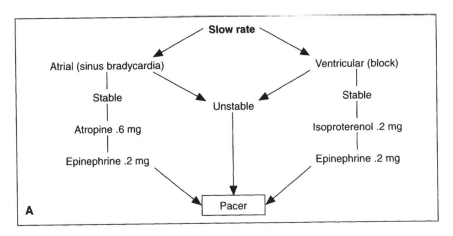

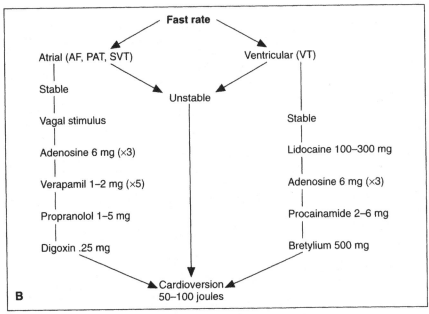

FIGURE 2-12. (A) Treatment of slow arrhythmias (B) treatment of fast arrhythmias. (AF = atrial fibrillation; PAT = paroxysmal atrial tachycardia; SVT = supraventricular tachycardia; VT = ventricular tachycardia.)

Monographs and Reviews

Camm AJ, Garratt CJ. Adenosine and supraventricular tachycardia. N Engl J Med 1991;325:1621–30.
A thorough review of the literature on adenosine and the rationale for using adenosine as the first drug of choice for the treatment of atrial tachycardias.

Dantzker DR. Cardiopulmonary physiology in critical care. Orlando, FL: Grune & Stratton, 1986.
This multiauthored textbook contains some excellent sections on hemodynamics and cardiopulmonary interactions in critical care.

Geddes LA and Baker LE, eds., Principles of applied biomedical instrumentation, 2nd ed. New York: Wiley, 1968.
A standard reference describing the principles and specific details of pressure and flow monitoring.

Harken AH. Cardiac arrhythmias. In: Holcroft J, ed. Care of the surgical patient. New York: Scientific American Medicine, 1991.
This is a multiauthored textbook on critical care published by the American College of Surgeons Committee on Pre- and Postoperative Care. The chapter on arrhythmias is one of the most practical and concise reviews of this topic.

Landis EM, Pappenheimer JR. Exchange of substances through capillary walls. In: Handbook of physiology: circulation (vol II). Baltimore: American Physiological Society, 1983:961–1034.
A review of transcapillary flux by the modern experts.

Moore FD. Metabolic care of the surgical patient. Philadelphia: Saunders, 1956.
This classic text is the standard reference describing body fluid compartments and transcapillary fluid kinetics in surgical and critically ill patients.

Scharf SM, Cassidy SS. Heart lung interactions in health and disease (vol 42, Lung Biology in Health and Disease). New York: Dekker, 1989.
This multiauthored monograph is the most complete single reference on cardiopulmonary interactions.

Selected Reports

DeSilva RA, Graboys TB, Podrid PJ, Lown B. Cardioversion and defibrillation. Am Heart J 1980;100:881–95.
Lown was the originator of the coronary care unit and developed DC defibrillation and cardioversion.

Fick A. On the measurement of the blood quantity in the ventricles of the heart. In: Proceedings of the Physiological, Medical Society of Wurzburg, July 9, 1870.
This is the original report of the "pencil experiment" describing the Fick axiom and Fick equation for cardiac output measurement.

Hamilton WF, Riley RL, Attyah AM, et al. Comparison of the Fick and dye injection methods of measuring the cardiac output in man. Am J Physiol 1948;153:309–16.

Hamilton adapted the dye dilution method originally described by Stewart many years before to measure cardiac output. This paper describes the collaboration between Hamilton and the Cournand-Richards group, who were developing the technique of cardiac catheterization. This collaboration resulted in the comparison of the Fick and dye dilution methods.

Hansen PD, Coffey SC, Lewis FR. The effects of adrenergic agents on oxygen delivery and oxygen consumption in normal dogs. J Trauma 1994;37:283–93.

One of many studies that shows the primary effect of catecholamines on systemic oxygen consumption.

Ognibene FP, Parker MM, Natanson C, et al. Depressed left ventricular performance: response to volume infusion in patients with sepsis and septic shock. Chest 1988;93:903–15.

This clinical study defines the hemodynamic events that take place in septic shock, including the response to volume infusion.

Sarnoff SJ. Myocardiac contractility as described by ventricular function curves; observations on Starling's law of the heart. Physiol Rev 1955;35:107–25.

Sarnoff provided the bridge from the laboratory setting to bedside practice.

Starling EH. The Linacre lecture on the law of the heart (Cambridge University, 1915). London: Longmans, Green, 1918.

The original description of Starling's law of the heart.

Swan HJC, Ganz W, Forrester JS, et al. Catheterization of the heart in man with the use of a flow directed balloon tipped catheter. N Engl J Med 1970;283:447–51.

The original description of the Swan-Ganz catheter.

Vincent JL, Preiser JC. Inotropic agents. New Horizons 1993;1:137–44.

This review published in the Society of Critical Care Medicine monograph series New Horizons defines the hemodynamic abnormalities in septic shock and the rationale for and results of many of the proposed treatments, including inotropic and alpha-adrenergic agents.

3

Respiratory Physiology and Pathophysiology

In the intensive care unit (ICU), the respiratory system commands an amount of attention and concern that is disproportionate to that commanded by other organ systems. Respiratory failure is the most common organ system failure in any ICU. Careful management is necessary to prevent respiratory failure in patients with normal lung function. Subconsciously we consider acute failure of the heart, kidneys, or liver to be an act of God, but acute respiratory failure somehow always seems like our fault—something we could have prevented or at least treated more successfully. The management of severe respiratory failure can become complex. The treatment itself, used to the extreme, is very damaging to the lung and requires a bit of art in addition to a lot of science.

The terms used to describe the respiratory system have precise definitions that are often overlapping and semisynonymous, and are frequently used incorrectly. Respiration is the overall process involved in oxygen getting from the atmosphere to the cells and combining with substrate and the resultant CO_2 returning to the atmosphere. Hence *respiration* might refer to gas exchange in the lungs, in the peripheral tissues, or at the mitochondrial or molecular level. Pulmonary respiration has two components: ventilation and gas exchange. Ventilation is the process of moving gas to and from the alveoli through the conducting airways and is synonymous with breathing. Everyone agrees on the definition of a breath, but a breath can be further described as a tidal breath, a vital capacity breath, a yawn, or a sigh, or as assisted or controlled. Pressure is needed for breathing to take place, and the pressure is described relative to the atmospheric pressure, but when pressure is discussed in relationship to volume, the inflating pressure is always considered positive, whether it is negative relative to the atmosphere or not. The interrelationships between gas volumes and intrathoracic pressure are lumped under the term *pulmonary mechanics*. The concept of gas exchange is easy to understand, but it is often forgotten that the processes related to

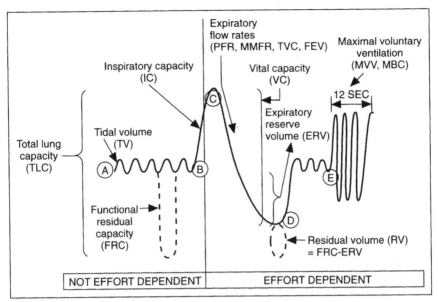

FIGURE 3-1. Lung volumes are measured by having the patient breathe in and out from a spirometer that measures volume changes. Flow and volume spirometry is commonly referred to as *pulmonary function tests*. (ERV = expiratory reserve volume; FEV = forced expiratory volume; MBC = maximum breathing capacity; MMFR = maximal mid-expiratory flow rate; PFR = peak flow rate; TVC = timed vital capacity.) (From: Bartlett RH. Posttraumatic pulmonary insufficiency. In: Cooper P, Nyhus L, eds. Surgery annual, 1971. New York: Appleton-Century-Crofts, 1971.)

CO_2 excretion (breathing) are quite different from the processes involved in oxygenation (ventilation-perfusion [$\dot{V}/\dot{Q}$] matching). Finally, the mechanical ventilator is such a large, obvious, and potentially dangerous apparatus that the process of mechanical ventilation is overemphasized in the management of respiratory failure, when attention might be better paid to the simpler but more important issues such as patient position, fluid balance, nutrition, and the treatment of anemia. In this chapter we discuss normal and abnormal pulmonary respiration and use the principles involved to define an algorithm for the prevention and management of pulmonary respiratory failure.

Pulmonary Mechanics

The interrelationships of the gas volumes and pressures involved with ventilation are referred to as *pulmonary mechanics*. Normal lung volumes are measured by spirometry, as shown in Figure 3-1. Tidal volume, inspiratory capacity, total lung capacity (TLC), and functional residual capacity (FRC) are

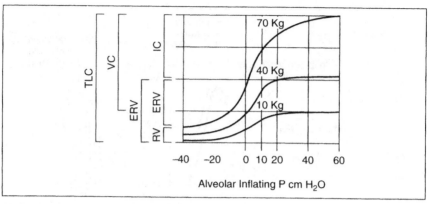

FIGURE 3-2. Volume-pressure curves. Normal lung volumes for subjects of 10, 40, and 70 kg are shown. Static lung volumes for the 70-kg subject are shown. Notice that full inflation of alveoli to total lung capacity (*TLC*) occurs at 40 cm H_2O for all sizes of subjects. (IC = inspiratory capacity; ERV = expiratory reserve volume; PRC = functional residual capacity; P = pressure; RV = residual volume; VC = vital capacity.)

not effort dependent, and hence can be measured in any patient who is breathing spontaneously or who is on a mechanical ventilator. The vital capacity (synonymous with forced expiratory volume [FEV]) is the amount of gas that a patient can exhale with maximum effort after a maximal inspiratory effort. The amount of gas that can be forcibly exhaled in 1 second (FEV_1), or fractions thereof, is an indirect measure of expiratory flow. In critically ill patients, determination of the FRC requires measurement with a relatively inert gas such as helium or with nitrogen during the breathing of 100% oxygen. The method is cumbersome, and therefore FRC is not commonly measured in the ICU, even though it is by far the most important of the lung volumes. Residual volume is not actually measured but is the difference between the expiratory reserve volume and the FRC.

The amount of gas volume that moves into or out of the lungs for a given amount of inflating or deflating pressure is referred to as *pulmonary compliance*. Compliance is usually expressed as a single number (X cc/cm H_2O), but this shorthand approach can be quite misleading. To understand and describe compliance it is necessary to compare volume and pressure relationships throughout an entire breath, which is done by plotting volume on the ordinate against pressure on the abscissa, thereby generating a compliance curve as shown in Figure 3-2. In this figure, expiratory or *de*flation volume-pressure curves are drawn for three normal subjects of different sizes. In each curve the patient has inhaled to TLC with an inflating pressure of 60 cm H_2O, then the pressure has been measured continuously as the patient exhales. Exhalation is a passive act between an inflating pressure of 60 cm H_2O and atmospheric pressure, then active exhalation is required

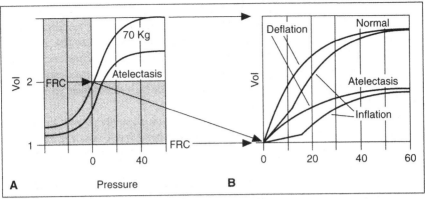

FIGURE 3-3. Volume-pressure curves in a normal 70-kg man, and the same man with atelectasis. By showing the end-expiratory volume as zero for each breath, the single breath compliance curve makes the smaller atelectatic lung appear stiffer. **A.** Compliance curves representing *deflation* from total lung capacity are shown for a normal 70 kg person and the same person with loss of alveolar volume because of atelectasis. The slope (compliance) is nearly the same for both curves, but TLC and FRC are decreased with atelectasis. Usually only the right upper quadrant of this graph is displayed, as in Fig B. **B.** The same deflation compliance curves as in A, but end expiration for each breath is plotted as zero volume, rather than true FRC. This makes the slope flatter, and the lung appears to be "stiffer." The *inflation* side of the volume-pressure curve is added to the deflation curves. In this example the inflation curve for atelectasis shows little alveolar recruitment until 16 cm H$_2$O is applied. (*FRC* = functional residual capacity.)

between atmospheric pressure and -40 cm H$_2$O in these examples. If the *in*flation half of the volume-pressure curve were shown for these normal subjects, it would be almost the same but shifted slightly to the right. Notice that full inflation of the alveoli to TLC occurs at about 40 cm H$_2$O for a single normal alveolus or a million alveoli, so that the shape of the volume-pressure curve is the same for all subjects; only the TLC and FRC are different. The compliance curve for a 70-kg adult who has undergone a left pneumonectomy would look the same as the normal compliance curve for a 40-kg child. The same would be true if the 70-kg adult lost half of his or her alveolar volume because of atelectasis, pneumonia, or edema. The concept of the functional lung being smaller (not "stiffer") is essential in the understanding and management of severe respiratory failure with a mechanical ventilator.

This concept is described in Figure 3-3. When the full volume-pressure curve is graphed out, it is easy to see how the decrease in FRC and TLC makes the lung "smaller" in the setting of atelectasis. The normal alveoli are inflated and the atelectactic alveoli are not. However, in clinical practice the full compliance curve is not displayed and the FRC is not measured. Instead, the compliance curve is displayed with the beginning and end point being atmospheric pressure and the FRC during each breath, rather than related to normal FRC. Therefore it appears that the compliance curve is flatter when alveolar volume is missing, and there is a tendency to say that the lung has become "stiffer." At present there is no practical way to readjust the volume baseline for shifting FRCs during breath-to-breath or minute-to-minute testing, so the artifact created by this problem must be understood in order to interpret bedside compliance curves.

What is the best way to measure the compliance curves shown in Figures 3-2 and 3-3? The simplest way is to inflate the lung from atmospheric pressure to TLC (either by voluntary effort or by a mechanical ventilator), then cap the airway, have the subject relax completely, and measure pressure at the mouth. This is referred to as *static compliance measurement*. It takes about 1 second for pressure at the mouth to come into equilibrium with the intrathoracic pressure. For our 70-kg adult the pressure at TLC is approximately 40 cm H_2O and the inspiratory capacity is about 2800 cc, so the static compliance is 70 cc/cm H_2O, or 1 cc/cm H_2O/kg. Actually this would be best described as "static pulmonary compliance at TLC." If we gradually allowed exhalation to take place but capped the airway and measured pressure every few hundred cubic centimeters, we would define several points on the deflation compliance curve that would ultimately allow us to plot the entire curve. This method is referred to as *quasistatic compliance testing*. A simpler method of defining the entire curve is to measure pressure at the airway (or in the thorax itself) continuously during deflation and plot the volume versus the pressure; this would result in the deflation curve shown in Figure 3-3. Notice that the normal lung is most compliant at pressures close to the atmospheric pressure, so that, if we expressed compliance at 10 cm H_2O of inflating pressure (rather than at 40 cm H_2O), we would find that the inflating volume is 1400 cc and the compliance is 2 cc/cm H_2O/kg.

When a patient is on a mechanical ventilator, volume, pressure, and flow are all controlled so that pulmonary mechanics can be measured and manipulated. The foregoing discussion of pulmonary mechanics actually refers to a pressure measured in the chest (by an intraesophageal manometer or by an intrapleural or intraesophageal monitor) while volume is measured at the mouth. Although this can be done in a ventilated patient, the common practice is to measure both the volume and the pressure at the mouth or at some other point closer to the mechanical ventilator. This practice introduces several variables and artifacts such as pressure gradients between the intrapleural space and the measuring site as well as compression and expansion volumes related to the machine and conduit tubing; in addition, the expiratory pressure may be intentionally elevated for patient management (positive end-expiratory pressure [PEEP]). When compliance is measured and reported in this fashion, it is referred to as *effective compliance*, meaning that the pressures and volumes are measured at the endotracheal tube or on the ventilator, taking all these variables into account. Hence, if our 70-kg patient has atelectasis and is on a mechanical ventilator set at an inspiratory plateau pressure of 30 cm H_2O with 10 cm H_2O of PEEP resulting in a tidal volume of 700 cc, we would say that the effective compliance is 700 cc/20 cm H_2O, or 35 cc/cm H_2O, or 0.5 cc/cm H_2O/kg.

The relationship of gas flow to pressure is referred to as *pulmonary resistance*. Resistance physiology is the major issue in the management of small-airway disease or bronchospasm, and bronchodilator drugs are titrated to minimize pulmonary resistance. The actual measurement of flow for these purposes is achieved with a sensitive gas flowmeter attached at the mouth or at the level of the endotracheal tube. This device is called a *pneumotachygraph*. Integrating flow with time yields the volume, and pneumotachygraphs are often used as volume measurement devices in studies of pulmonary mechanics.

Effect of Position on Pulmonary Mechanics

All of the foregoing discussion about normal pulmonary mechanics is based on the mechanics in normal subjects tested in a sitting position. However, most of our patients are supine. In the supine position the stomach, liver, spleen, and other abdominal viscera press down on the posterior half of the diaphragm, physically compressing the lung bases and requiring extra effort on the part of the diaphragm to "lift up" the abdominal viscera off of the compressed lung during contraction. (Remember, at FRC most of the diaphragm is oriented in a coronal rather than a transverse plane.) Therefore both the FRC and TLC are considerably decreased in a subject who is supine rather than sitting. In the same subject when standing, the weight of the abdominal viscera actually pulls down on the diaphragm (the same is true in a kneeling, prone subject). Therefore the FRC is the highest in the standing or prone, kneeling position. In a subject lying completely prone, the viscera press on the smaller anterior parts of the lung bases and abdominal motion is limited, so that FRC and TLC are slightly less than they are in a subject in the sitting position. All of these relationships are diagrammed in Figure 3-4.

The effect of a patient's position on lung volume affects lung compliance. The FRC is smaller when the patient is supine, so greater pressure is required to achieve full inflation. Moreover, force is required to lift the weight of the abdominal viscera. The net effect is that compliance is considerably lower in a supine subject compared to the same subject sitting or standing. This becomes important when one is trying to wean patients from mechanical ventilation to resume spontaneous breathing. Much less effort is needed when the patient is sitting or standing (or, for that matter, kneeling) than when supine. The same principles must be considered when one is trying to recruit atelectatic alveoli. Atelectasis almost always occurs in the posterior aspects of the lung, partly because of the effects of that posture, and it is always easier to inflate collapsed posterior alveoli with the patient sitting, standing, or prone.

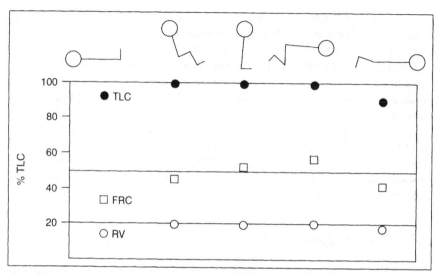

FIGURE 3-4. Lung volumes measured at various body positions. The abdominal viscera compress the lung, decreasing the functional residual capacity (*FRC*) in the supine position. (TLC = total lung capacity; RV = residual volume.) Adapted from Agostoni E, Mead J. Statics of the respiratory system. In: Fenn W, Rahn H, (eds). Handbook of physiology: Respiration, Pt 3, vol 1, 1964. Washington, DC: American Physiological Society.

In acute respiratory failure the cause of decreased compliance is almost always associated with a decrease in the FRC (see Figure 3-3). This decreased FRC is due to the loss of alveoli, either because they have collapsed or are filled with fluid but still perfused with blood. One way of managing ventilation in this circumstance is to stop expiration when the pressure is still positive (PEEP). For example, a PEEP set at 10 cm H_2O maintains the inflation of alveoli that otherwise might close at lower end-expiratory pressures. When this happens, the functional lung is larger and the entire compliance curve shifts back toward the left.

Several measurements must be performed to determine whether the positive airway pressure is recruiting collapsed alveoli or simply distending normal alveoli (Figure 3-5). When collapsed alveoli are being reinflated, compliance improves, dead space ventilation decreases, cardiac output is unaffected, oxygenation improves at the same ventilator settings as shunt decreases, and the risk of air leak is minimal. These principles and measurements must be kept in mind during the management of the patient on a mechanical ventilator.

Lung damage can be caused by a high airway pressure, so that overdistention as shown in Figure 3-2 is not merely inefficient but actually detrimental. Because the most normal areas of lung have the best compliance, they are the most vulnerable to overdistention, thereby contributing to the steady

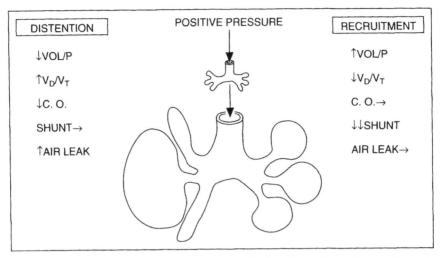

FIGURE 3-5. When inflating pressure is applied to the collapsed lung, the goal is equal inflation of all alveoli (recruitment), but unequal inflation (distention) is possible. (C.O. = cardiac output; VOL/P = volume-pressure ratio; V_D/V_T = dead space-to-tidal volume ratio.) (From: Bartlett RH, Respiratory care of the surgical patient. Surg Clin North Am, Vol. 62, No. 6, 1980.)

progression of lung dysfunction in patients ventilated at a high peak pressure. Every effort should be made to keep the peak inspiratory pressure under 40 cm H_2O, and preferably lower.

Definitions and formulas related to pulmonary mechanics are given in Table 3-1.

Gas Exchange

Gas exchange refers to oxygen and CO_2 transfer that takes place between the ventilating gas and the blood. It is best to consider the exchange of these two gases separately. The definitions and formulas related to gas exchange are given in Tables 1-1 and 3-2. The methods of measuring and describing oxygen content in blood are discussed in detail in Chapter 1 and diagrammed in Figures 1-2 and 1-3. The partial pressure of oxygen (P_{O_2}) of dry air is 20.9% of the barometric pressure, or 157 mm Hg at sea level. By the time inhaled gas reaches the alveoli, the partial pressure of water vapor is 47 mm Hg and the P_{O_2} is 149 mm Hg. The P_{O_2} in the pulmonary capillary blood is approximately 40 mm Hg, so at the first instant of inspiration there is a gradient of 109 mm Hg between the alveolus and the capillary blood and oxygen diffuses across the alveolar membrane into the blood in response to this gradient. During the rest of the breath, oxygen diffuses out of the alveolus into the blood, so that at the end of a normal breath (that is, after 5

TABLE 3-1. Pulmonary Mechanics

Abbreviation	Definition/Formula	Normal Value
TLC	Total lung capacity	80 cc/kg
FRC	Functional residual capacity	40 cc/kg
IC	Inspiratory capacity	40 cc/kg
ERV	Expiratory reserve volume	30 cc/kg
RV	Residual volume	10 cc/kg
V_T	Tidal volume	5 cc/kg
$\dot{V}_E$	Minute ventilation (exhaled)	100 cc/kg/min
$\dot{V}_A$	Alveolar ventilation	60 cc/kg/min
V_D	Dead space	cc = weight in lbs
PIP	Peak inspiratory pressure	10 cm H_2O tidal, 40 cm H_2O max
EIP (on ventilator)*	End-inspiratory (plateau) pressure	less than PIP
EEP	End-expiratory pressure	0 cm H_2O
Compliance	V_T/EIP	2 cc/cm H_2O/kg
Effective compliance	V_T/EIP − PEEP on ventilator	1 cc/cm H_2O/kg
Resistance	Inspiratory flow/pressure	—
V_D/V_T	$\dfrac{PaCO_2 - PECO_2}{PaCO_2}$	0.33

CO_2 = partial pressure in mixed expired gas; $PaCO_2$ = arterial CO_2 pressure; $PECO_2$ = mixed expired CO_2; PEEP = positive end-expiratory pressure.
*Normal EIP value depends on ventilator settings.

TABLE 3-2. Respiration

Abbreviation	Definition/Formula	Normal Value
CaO_2	Oxygen content, arterial	20 cc/dL
CvO_2	Oxygen content, venous	16 cc/dL
PAO_2	Alveolar PO_2 = [(P_B − P_{H_2O}) × FiO_2] − $PaCO_2$	100 mm Hg (air), 673 mm Hg (FiO_2 = 1.0)
$AaDO_2$	Alveolar-arterial O_2 gradient: PAO_2 − PaO_2	10 mm Hg (air), 70 mm Hg (FiO_2 = 1.0)
PaO_2/FiO_2	Oxygen index (bedside shorthand)	500
CcO_2	Theoretical maximal CaO_2 at known FiO_2	22 cc/dL at FiO_2 and Hgb of 15 g/dL
% Shunt	$\dfrac{CcO_2 - CaO_2}{CcO_2 - CvO_2}$	5%

FiO_2 = fraction of inspired oxygen; Hgb = hemoglobin; $PaCO_2$ = arterial CO_2 pressure; P_B = barometric pressure; P_{H_2O} = 47 mm Hg at 37°C.

or 6 seconds) the PO_2 in both the alveolus and the capillary blood exiting the alveolus is about 90 mm Hg. This is true for an alveolus in the middle of the lung, and if all the alveoli had equal ventilation and perfusion the arterial PO_2 (PaO_2) would be the average PO_2 during the breath, or about 115 mm Hg. However, in a sitting subject, alveoli at the apex of the lung have relatively low blood flow and blood entering the pulmonary veins from those alveoli has an average PO_2 of approximately 120 mm Hg. On the other hand, alveoli at the base of the lung have more blood flow than ventilation and the PO_2 in the blood exiting those alveoli is approximately 80 mm Hg. Blood from all of

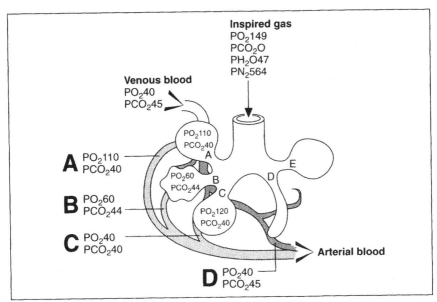

FIGURE 3-6. Normal venous blood (PO_2 = 40 mm Hg, PCO_2 = 45 mm Hg) perfusing five different areas of lung representing different ventilation-perfusion relationships. (See text for explanation of A to E.) (From Bartlett, RH. Posttraumatic pulmonary insufficiency. In: Cooper P, Nyhus L, eds. Surgery annual, 1971. New York: Appleton-Century-Crofts, 1971.)

these alveoli mixes in the left ventricle, so that the resultant PaO_2 in a normal person who is seated and breathing air is approximately 90 mm Hg. During vigorous exercise, ventilation and perfusion both increase and equalize, so that the Po_2 in a subject during exercise while breathing air is normally approximately 110 mm Hg. Another factor contributing to the normal end-tidal gradient between alveolar gas and arterial blood oxygen is the fact that about 3% of the blood arriving in the left atrium comes from the bronchial circulation or thebesian veins and is not fully oxygenated (the normal "anatomic" shunt).

Increasing the fraction of inspired oxygen (FiO_2) increases the gradient for oxygen transfer, but the same principles of equilibration during a single breath apply. Therefore, even though the Po_2 of inhaled gas while breathing 100% oxygen is 713 mm Hg and the Po_2 of end-tidal alveolar gas is 673 mm Hg, the normal PaO_2 during 100% oxygen breathing is approximately 600 mm Hg.

Oxygen transfer in the lung and the causes of hypoxemia are depicted in Figure 3-6. Under normal conditions, red blood cells in the pulmonary capillaries become fully saturated and oxygen dissolves in the plasma, resulting in a blood Po_2 of 100 mm Hg (after coming into equilibrium at the end of a resting expiration) and an arterial oxygen saturation (SaO_2) of 100% (see Figure 3-6, A). This equilibration may be disturbed by hypoventilation in

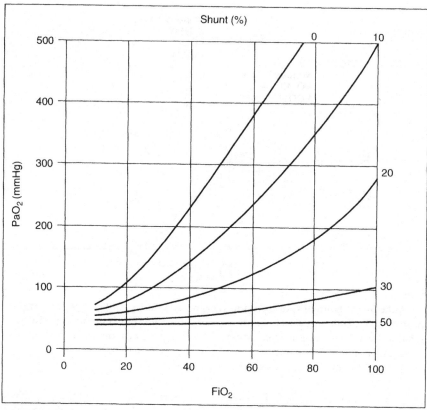

FIGURE 3-7. Oxygenation measured as PaO_2 at various levels of transpulmonary shunt and FiO_2.

relation to the perfusion ($\dot{V}/\dot{Q}$ mismatch; see Figure 3-6, *B*), by diffusion block caused by interstitial fibrosis (see Figure 3-6, *C*), or by the perfusion of nonventilated alveoli (simply the extreme of hypoventilation, see Figure 3-6, *D*). Diffusion block and $\dot{V}/\dot{Q}$ mismatch can be almost completely overcome by having the patient breathe 100% oxygen, hence the hypoxemia that occurs during exposure to a high alveolar Po_2 is caused by total $\dot{V}/\dot{Q}$ mismatch, so-called transpulmonary shunting or venous admixture. Under normal conditions, approximately 5% of the blood entering the left atrium has been shunted away form the pulmonary capillaries, either as a result of bronchial nutritive blood flow or through thebesian veins opening directly into the left side of the heart. This phenomenon, combined with the normal minor $\dot{V}/\dot{Q}$ mismatch associated with breathing at rest and positional effects on pulmonary blood flow, result in the fact that the normal PaO_2 is 90 mm Hg and the normal SaO_2 is 99%. The extent to which various degrees of transpulmonary shunting affect arterial oxygenation is shown in Figure 3-7.

The shunt fraction is actually calculated by assuming that the blood in the capillaries in those alveolocapillary units that are functioning normally is fully saturated and equilibrated with end-tidal gas. The oxygen content in these theoretically perfectly normal units is calculated based on the assumption that the blood is fully saturated and fully equilibrated at the end-tidal alveolar Po_2. For example, if the subject is breathing 100% oxygen and the arterial CO_2 pressure ($PaCO_2$) is 40 mm Hg, it is assumed that the Po_2 in the end-tidal alveolar gas and in the blood perfusing those alveoli is 673 mm Hg at sea level. Therefore the oxygen content in these theoretically optimal units is determined by the following formula: (hemoglobin level × 100% × 1.36) + (0.003 × 673). In addition, it is assumed that blood passing through areas of transpulmonary shunt is identical to venous blood. With these assumptions, the fraction of blood passing through the shunt ($\dot{Q}s/\dot{Q}t$) can be calculated as follows:

$$\frac{\dot{Q}s}{\dot{Q}t} = \frac{CcO_2 - CaO_2}{CcO_2 - CvO_2},$$

where $CaCO_2$ is the arterial oxygen content, CcO_2 is the oxygen content of blood leaving the capillaries of normal alveoli, and CvO_2 is the venous oxygen content.

Sampling arterial and venous blood and going through all the calculations is somewhat cumbersome, so the shunt fraction is often estimated from a graph such as that shown in Figure 3-7. Obviously the effect of the venous blood content on the shunt calculation is considerable; therefore, if oxygen delivery is decreased because of low cardiac output or a low hemoglobin level, venous saturation will decline, decreasing the calculated shunt fraction. This is not a mathematical artifact but reflects the fact that autoregulation causes pulmonary blood flow to be diverted away from nonventilated areas at a low cardiac output, but this effect is overridden at higher cardiac outputs, resulting in more shunting (Figure 3-8). The shunt fraction can be calculated at any level of FiO_2, but such a calculation includes components of diffusion block and $\dot{V}/\dot{Q}$ mismatch when the FiO_2 is less than 1.0. The level of lung dysfunction can be similarly estimated by calculating the alveolar arterial (Aa) gradient for oxygen ($AaDO_2$) or the PaO_2 divided by FiO_2. The Aa gradient is calculated as follows:

$$AaDO_2 = ([P_B - P_{H_2O}] \times FiO_2) - PaCO_2 - PaO_2,$$

where P_B is the barometric pressure, P_{H_2O} is 47 mm Hg at 37°C, and assuming that the alveolar PCO_2 is identical to the $PaCO_2$ (not necessarily true). With these assumptions, the normal Aa gradient is approximately 10 mm Hg when breathing air and 70 mm Hg when breathing 100% oxygen. Aa gradient greater than 500 corresponds to approximately 30% transpulmonary shunt.

The PaO_2 over FiO_2 calculation is simply bedside shorthand for characterizing the Aa gradient without all the calculations. The normal value is 500,

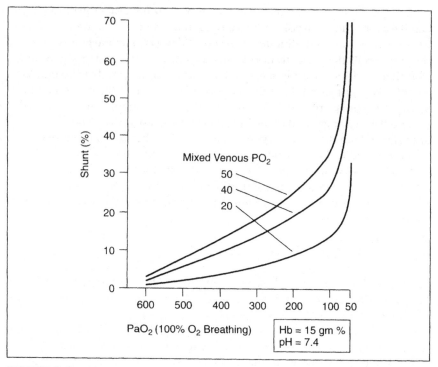

FIGURE 3-8. The higher the mixed venous oxygen pressure (PO_2), the greater the shunt. This is because blood flow through nonventilated lung increases with increasing cardiac output; increasing cardiac output is reflected as a higher venous saturation. (PaO_2 = arterial oxygen pressure.) (From: Bartlett RH. Posttraumatic pulmonary insufficiency. In: Cooper P, Nyhus L, eds. Surgery annual, 1971. New York: Appleton-Century-Crofts, 1971.)

and a value of 100 corresponds to a 30% shunt. These four methods of characterizing lung dysfunction based on oxygenation are diagrammed in Figure 3-9.

Before leaving the discussion of oxygenation, it should be noted that the interruption of blood flow to alveoli has no effect on oxygenation, except by diverting blood flow to all the other areas of lung (see Figure 3-6, *E*). If the remainder of the lung is basically normal, then the occlusion of pulmonary arteries should have no effect on oxygenation. However, we all have encountered patients with a pulmonary embolism who become hypoxic. This occurs because blood flow must increase through areas of $\dot{V}/\dot{Q}$ mismatch and shunting, or right atrial pressure increases to the point where right-to-left shunting occurs through the foramen ovale, or the residence time of red blood cells in pulmonary capillaries becomes so brief that the time for oxygenation is inadequate, or any combination of these causes. Of these causes, the last one

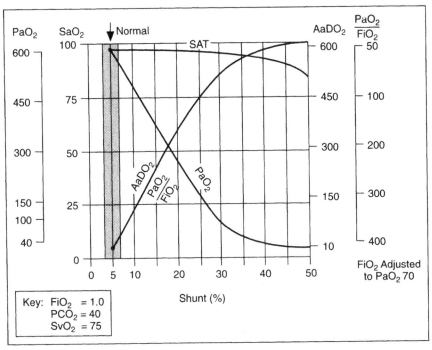

FIGURE 3-9. Four methods of describing lung dysfunction based on lung oxygenation. For the curves describing saturation (*SAT*) and PaO$_2$, it is assumed that FiO$_2$ = 1.0, PaCO$_2$ = 40 mm Hg, and the venous oxygen saturation (*SvO$_2$*) = 75%. For the curve describing the alveolar-arterial gradient (*AaDO$_2$*) and PaO$_2$/FiO$_2$ ratio, it is assumed that FiO$_2$ is adjusted to maintain PaO$_2$ at 70 mm Hg and arterial oxygen saturation (*SaO$_2$*) at 95%.

can be largely corrected with supplemental oxygen, raising the gradient for oxygen diffusion in the pulmonary capillaries.

CO$_2$ Kinetics: Ventilation and Metabolism

As mentioned previously, oxygen uptake across the lung is related to V̇/Q̇ relationships and the alveolar Po$_2$. CO$_2$ excretion, on the other hand, is related to the amount of ventilation. Because CO$_2$ is much more diffusible than oxygen and because a small amount of hyperventilation excretes a large amount of CO$_2$, the limiting factors controlling oxygenation and CO$_2$ removal are quite different.

The total amount of CO$_2$ produced by systemic metabolism is roughly equivalent to the amount of oxygen consumed (100 to 120 cc/m^2/min, or 200 cc/min in a typical adult). The ratio between CO$_2$ produced and oxygen consumed is called the *respiratory quotient* (R or RQ) and varies slightly depending on the foodstuff being metabolized.

Measurement of CO_2

CO_2 in gas is measured with an infrared spectrophotometer. The spectrophotometer is calibrated against the known standard to read out as the percentage of CO_2 or partial pressure of CO_2 (P_{CO_2}). The P_{CO_2} in gas can also be measured by injecting the gas to be tested into a conventional blood gas machine containing a CO_2 electrode. The P_{CO_2} in blood (or gas) is measured by a CO_2 electrode described by Severinghaus. The electrode consists of a pH electrode surrounded by an electrolyte solution and covered by a gas-permeable membrane. The electrode is placed in the test solution, and CO_2 equilibrates across the membrane, causing a change in pH that is registered as a voltage change. When this electrode is calibrated against known standards, the P_{CO_2} can be measured. Blood gas machines contain a Clark electrode, a Severinghaus electrode, and an uncovered pH electrode. Thus, the primary measurements are P_{O_2}, P_{CO_2}, and pH, respectively. The temperature is maintained at 37°C. Based on these four controlled or measured variables, the saturation and bicarbonate and buffer base deviation are calculated. If the hemoglobin level is known, then the oxygen content can be calculated and the bicarbonate level can be calculated more exactly by taking into account the effects of carbamino compounds. Most blood gas machines in current use purge the blood sample with cleaning solution and automatically inject a calibrating solution, then print out the results, which include three actual measurements, a host of calculations, and even a professional sounding interpretation ("Moderate hypoxemia with hypocapnia and mild respiratory alkalosis. This pattern suggests hypoxemia with compensatory hyperventilation.").

CO_2 production is increased or decreased by each of the factors that affects $\dot{V}_{O_2}$. Most of the CO_2 in blood is present as bicarbonate ion that cannot change quickly (somewhat analogous to the total blood hemoglobin level or red blood cell mass in relationship to the oxygen content). However, the metabolically produced CO_2 is mostly present in the form of dissolved CO_2, which is added to the blood in the peripheral tissues and excreted in the lung. The relationships between CO_2 content, bicarbonate concentration, and the dissolved CO_2 are shown in Figure 3-10. Notice that the arteriovenous concentration difference for CO_2 is 5 cc/dL, the same as that for oxygen. In a steady state the amount of CO_2 excreted through the lung is exactly equal to the amount of CO_2 produced in peripheral tissues. However, because the amount excreted is so easily influenced by minor changes in ventilation, the assurance of a steady state is particularly important when the volume of CO_2 produced is measured at the airway. The amount of CO_2 excreted is a function of the ventilation of perfused alveoli (that is, the

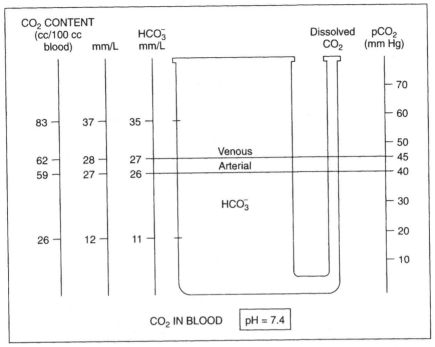

FIGURE 3-10. The distribution of CO_2 in blood. (From Bartlett RH. Posttraumatic pulmonary insufficiency. In: Cooper P, Nyhus L, eds. Surgery annual, 1971. New York: Appleton-Century-Crofts, 1971.)

alveolar ventilation per minute). The relationship between alveolar ventilation and CO_2 excretion is shown in Figure 3-11.

CO_2 Transfer in the Lung

The amount of CO_2 excreted is directly related to the alveolar ventilation, as already discussed. Even if 75% of the alveoli are not inflated, hyperventilation of the remaining 25% can maintain normocapnia in arterial blood, whereas profound hypoxemia will result from a 75% shunt regardless of the FiO_2 or the ventilation of remaining alveoli. These relationships are shown in Figure 3-12, again illustrating that oxygenation is a function of matching blood flow to inflated alveoli, whereas CO_2 excretion is a function of ventilation or hyperventilation of alveoli with some blood flow. In this example the shunt fraction is 50%. Pulmonary arterial blood has a saturation of 80%. Half the blood goes to the shunt and exits unchanged. The other half of the blood goes to inflated alveoli and becomes fully saturated, so that the resultant saturation is 90% with systemic hypoxemia at a Po_2 of 55 mm Hg. The same distribution of blood flow occurs with regard to CO_2 exchange, and

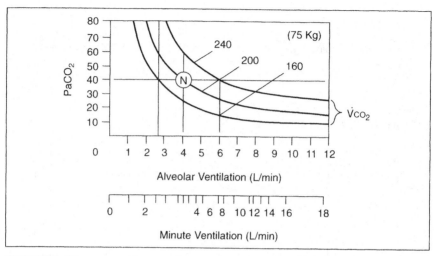

FIGURE 3-11. CO_2 excretion ($\dot{V}CO_2$) related to ventilation for a typical 75-kg adult. (N = normal.) (Adapted from: Nunn JF, ed. Applied respiratory physiology. London: Butterworths, 1969.)

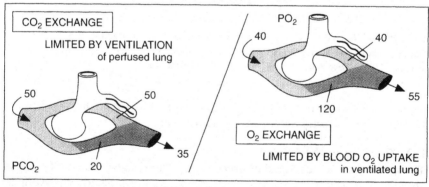

FIGURE 3-12. Oxygen and CO_2 exchange during shunt. (From Bartlett RH. Respiratory care of the surgical patient. Surg Clin North Am Vol. 62, No. 1, 1980.)

blood leaves the collapsed alveoli at a P_{CO_2} of 50 mm Hg. However, hyperventilation of the functional alveoli reduces the P_{CO_2} to 20 mm Hg, so that the resulting $PaCO_2$ is 35 mm Hg.

Oxygenation can be monitored continuously and on-line by measuring saturation either in blood or transcutaneously with a pulse oximeter. Unfortunately there is no effective way to measure the blood P_{CO_2} continuously. Several companies have developed micro–P_{CO_2} electrodes that are moderately effective, but electrical drift and thrombosis on the membrane limits reliability, and a measurement device that is not reliable is worse than no device at all. Consequently, currently on-line blood gas measurements are possible but impractical. Because the CO_2 in exhaled gas is in equilibrium with the P_{CO_2} in blood and because the P_{CO_2} can be measured with a spectrophotometer at the exact end of a normal breath (end-tidal measurements), this measurement of end-tidal CO_2 can be used to estimate the blood $PaCO_2$ continuously.

Normally the end-tidal CO_2 represents mixed alveolar gas that is in equilibrium with pulmonary capillary blood, hence with arterial blood. Therefore the end-tidal P_{CO_2} and the $PaCO_2$ should be almost identical. The respiratory center is keenly sensitive to the level of P_{CO_2}, such that the automatic rate and depth of breathing is regulated to maintain the $PaCO_2$ at 40 mm Hg. The end-tidal P_{CO_2} should be the same or just slightly less than $PaCO_2$. There is no way that the $PaCO_2$ can be lower than the end-tidal P_{CO_2}. If some of the end-tidal gas has not been in equilibrium with pulmonary capillary blood, this gas will not contain CO_2 and will cause the CO_2 to be diluted in end-tidal measurements, such that the end-tidal P_{CO_2} is lower than the $PaCO_2$. This situation will occur whenever there is a considerable amount of lung that is ventilated but not perfused (that is, dead space) and/or overventilated and minimally perfused, and/or some of the end-tidal gas represents inflation gas that is simply compressed and released, never having reached the alveoli. The latter situation inevitably occurs under any positive-pressure ventilation circumstance but only creates a significant end-tidal $PaCO_2$ gradient when the peak airway pressures are very high (more than 30 cm H_2O) and the compression volume is a significant component of each exhaled breath. The end-tidal P_{CO_2} measurement then becomes a very useful way of continuously monitoring $PaCO_2$ when the lung is nearly normal, such as when weaning a patient off a mechanical ventilator. In addition, the gradient between the end-tidal and arterial P_{CO_2}, when large, acts as an indirect measure of nonperfused alveoli or compression volume, or both. The details of end-tidal P_{CO_2} monitoring are diagrammed in Figure 3-13.

Pathophysiology of Respiratory Failure

The lung has a limited repertoire of ways to respond to injury. Regardless of the specific cause, pulmonary dysfunction can be classified under two headings, (1) alveolar collapse, partial or complete, that is, decreased FRC, and (2) pulmonary edema caused by high hydrostatic pressure or increased capillary permeability, or both.

Alveolar Collapse

A decrease in the FRC is caused by incomplete alveolar inflation related to (1) shallow breathing; (2) partial or complete airway occlusion, which may

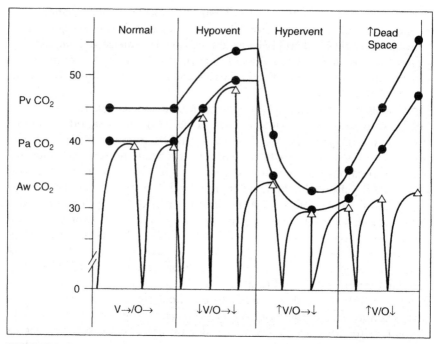

FIGURE 3-13. End-tidal CO_2 pressure monitoring. In this example, venous (*Pv*), arterial (*Pa*), and airway (*Aw*) PCO_2 are shown during various breathing patterns. The end-tidal CO_2 pressure is very close to the $PaCO_2$ as long as there is no dead space at the alveolar level. Increased alveolar level dead space (such as that caused by emphysematous bullae, honeycombing resulting from lung injury, or the exclusion of blood flow by fibrosis or low cardiac output) causes the end-tidal CO_2 pressure to be lower than the $PaCO_2$. (V/Q = ventilation-perfusion.)

be generalized (as in bronchospasm) or localized (as in gastric aspiration); (3) absorption atelectasis, which occurs when oxygen is substituted for nitrogen in the inspired gas; or (4) conditions in which air or fluid is occupying potential alveolar space in the chest, such as in the settings of pneumothorax, hemothorax, or pulmonary edema. Figure 3-14 lists the causes and effects of alveolar collapse.

The pulmonary arteriolar spasm that occurs in response to local hypoxia autoregulates pulmonary blood flow and maintains adequate gas exchange during alveolar collapse—up to a point. However, when the loss in ventilation exceeds the decrease in perfusion, a $\dot{V}/\dot{Q}$ mismatch occurs, which results in incomplete oxygenation of the blood perfusing that area of lung. The resultant hypoxemia stimulates an increased rate and depth of breathing, which may serve to reexpand the partially inflated area of lung. If it does not, the hypoxemia will continue but increased ventilation in other areas of lung will result in excess CO_2 excretion, hypocapnia, and respiratory alkalosis.

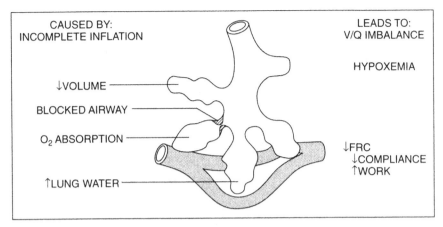

FIGURE 3-14. Causes and effects of alveolar collapse. (FRC = functional residual capacity; V/Q = ventilation-perfusion.) (From Bartlett RH. Respiratory care of the surgical patient. Surg Clin North Am Vol. 62, No. 1, 1980.)

This blood gas picture, hypoxemia with respiratory alkalosis, is the most common abnormality of gas exchange in ICU patients and is the hallmark of $\dot{V}/\dot{Q}$ imbalance.

Oxygenation of blood in the poorly ventilated area of lung can be improved by the increasing concentration of oxygen in the inspired gas. As long as the airways are pinhole patent and the alveoli are inflated at all, the hypoxemia of $\dot{V}/\dot{Q}$ imbalance can be reversed by the provision of supplemental oxygen. Of course this treats the symptom rather than the basic cause and may actually make the problems worse by compounding the absorption atelectasis, thus depriving the poorly ventilated area of nitrogen needed to hold the alveoli open. This may lead to total alveolar collapse. In this circumstance, blood perfusing the nonventilated area (transpulmonary shunt) will mix with blood from other areas of the lung, resulting in hypoxemia that does not abate significantly in response to the administration of oxygen.

The reasons for this are shown in Figure 3-12. Blood perfusing the atelectatic lung mixes with blood perfusing the more normal lung, resulting in a decrease in oxygenation and an increase in the blood CO_2 level. Increasing the FiO_2 to 1.0 may result in a large increase in Po_2 in the blood exiting the normal lung. However, the major increase in Po_2 is associated with a very small increase in oxygen content, as the oxygen that raises the Po_2 (from 100 to 500 mm Hg, for example) is the small amount dissolved in plasma. The oxygenation of arterial blood is an average of the oxygen content of blood from the two areas of lung, not an average of the Po_2. Therefore systemic hypoxia will persist regardless of the FiO_2. When this hypoxemic, hypercapnic blood reaches the respiratory center, the rate and depth of breathing are increased. This results in hyperventilation of the normal lung but no change in ventilation of the atelectatic lung. This hyperventilation has a minimal effect on the oxygenation of blood exiting from the normal lung for the reasons just outlined. However, it results in an excessive excretion of CO_2, leading to respiratory alkalosis, just as occurs in the setting of lesser degrees of $\dot{V}/\dot{Q}$ mismatch discussed earlier.

Aside from the effects on gas exchange, the loss of alveolar space produces changes in the volume-pressure relationships in the lung (that is, pulmonary mechanics). As shown in Figure 3-3, a decrease in FRC results in a shift in the volume-pressure relationship toward a condition of decreasing compliance. That is, more pressure is required to achieve the same degree of lung inflation. The pressure specified in this graph is the alveolar inflating pressure, or the transalveolar pressure. This pressure is plotted as positive if it serves to inflate alveoli, whether the relationship to atmospheric pressure is positive (as it is in mechanical ventilation) or negative (as it is in spontaneous breathing). This method of expressing volume-pressure relationships is a standard one and seems straightforward. However, it can become complex when a patient is breathing spontaneously while positive pressure is being applied to the airway. Remember that "negative" pressure applied to the pleural space by the diaphragm and "positive" pressure applied to the airway with a ventilator are additive from the standpoint of volume-pressure characteristics.

Pulmonary Edema

There are three causes of pulmonary edema: (1) increased hydrostatic pressure (left ventricular failure or gross fluid overload); (2) decreased plasma oncotic pressure (rarely a problem unless the concentration of plasma protein is very low); and (3) increased capillary permeability (Figure 3-15). When fluid begins to collect in the lung interstitium, it migrates to the loose areolar portions of the lung microanatomy that surround the small bronchioles and pulmonary arteries. Edema in these areas has the effect of narrowing bronchi and increasing resistance in the pulmonary vasculature. This decreases both ventilation and perfusion in the edematous area, but ventilation is often affected more than is blood flow, resulting in a decreased $\dot{V}/\dot{Q}$ ratio, with all of its attendant effects on gas exchange. As more fluid collects in the lung, it may compress alveoli and eventually flood into the alveoli, further decreasing the FRC and ultimately leading to transpulmonary shunting.

The interrelationships between lung edema, atelectasis, and gas exchange in ICU patients are often misunderstood. The amount of lung dysfunction (measured as a shunt, $\dot{V}/\dot{Q}$ imbalance, or decreased compliance) may parallel changes in the degree of pulmonary edema or may be totally unrelated (Figure 3-16). Under normal conditions there is a net efflux of "filtrate" across the pulmonary capillary bed at a rate of about 20 mL/hr. This fluid is entirely cleared from the lung by means of the lung lymphatics. When the amount of transcapillary filtrate increases for any reason, the rate of lymph

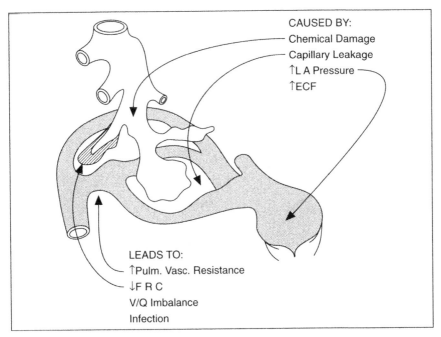

FIGURE 3-15. Causes and effects of pulmonary edema in acute respiratory failure. (ECF = extracellular fluid; FRC = functional residual capacity; LA = left atrial; V/Q = ventilation-perfusion.) (From Bartlett RH. Respiratory care of the surgical patient. Surg Clin North Am Vol. 62, No. 1, 1980.)

flow increases proportionately, with no net change in the amount of fluid in the lung interstitium. When the lymphatic drainage can no longer keep pace with the amount of transcapillary filtrate, fluid begins to accumulate in the interstitium. This process continues until the interstitial fluid space of the lung is increased by a factor of two or more, then alveolar flooding begins. If the amount of fluid in all the alveoli approaches the amount in the interstitium, this is incompatible with life. Pronounced changes in lung function do not occur until the level of interstitial water is grossly above normal, and at that point $\dot{V}/\dot{Q}$ mismatch begins. With slightly more transcapillary filtrate, alveolar flooding and shunting occur (Figure 3-17). With these relationships in mind, consider the effect of ventilator treatment: Increased airway pressure tends to hold alveoli open, spread out the space available for water accumulation, and overcome the effects of small bronchial occlusion (Figure 3-18). These effects are observed when there is minimal edema, right up to the time when the lung is filled with fluid. This is why positive airway pressure improves gas exchange in the setting of pulmonary edema. (Positive pressure does not affect the actual amount of edema in the lung, only its manifestations.) This discussion illustrates the point that edema affects pulmonary function only at the extreme, and even then minor changes in the

70 Critical Care Physiology

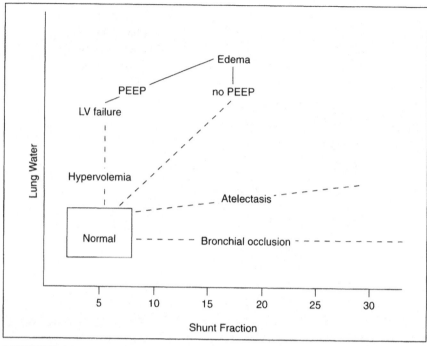

FIGURE 3-16. Shunt fraction related to the amount of edema in the lung. (LV = left ventricular; PEEP = positive end-expiratory pressure.)

amount of pulmonary water can lead to major changes in function. This fact, combined with the observation that any patients may have atelectasis for reasons unrelated to pulmonary edema, leads to confusion about and misunderstanding concerning this aspect of pathophysiology.

Recently Gattinoni has pointed out that the deleterious effects of interstitial edema are caused not only by swollen airways and alveolar filling but also by the simple fact that the weight of the edematous lung is compressing the dependent lung below it. This phenomenon became obvious when patients with diffuse interstitial edema resulting from adult respiratory distress syndrome (ARDS) were examined by computed tomographic (CT) scanning. Although the conventional anteroposterior chest x-ray study is said to show diffuse homogeneous fluid infiltrates throughout both lung fields, CT scans clearly show that the infiltrates are not diffuse or homogeneous at all, but rather consolidated in the most dependent areas of the lung. For most critically ill patients the dependent areas are the posterior areas because the patients are supine. Figure 3-19 shows the CT scan of a patient with ARDS. In the scan shown in Figure 3-19A, the patient is supine and the posterior consolidation involves almost a third of the lung. Blood flowing through this consolidated area does not participate in gas exchange and contributes to the transpulmonary shunting. The more anterior lung is relatively normal and accounts for some of the oxygenation and ample CO_2 clearance. Figure

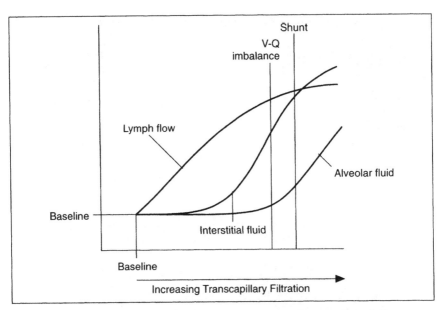

FIGURE 3-17. Alveolar fluid, interstitial fluid, and pulmonary lymph flow during progressive levels of pulmonary capillary leakage. (V-Q Imbal = ventilation-perfusion imbalance.) (From Bartlett RH. Respiratory care of the surgical patient. Surg Clin North Am Vol. 62, No. 1, 1980.)

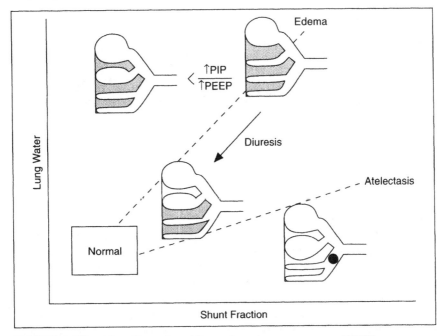

FIGURE 3-18. The effect of positive end-expiratory pressure (PEEP) on interstitial edema. (PIP = peak inspiratory pressure.) The shaded area represents increased lung water. Compare to Fig. 3.16.

72   Critical Care Physiology

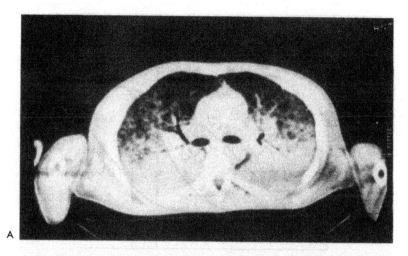

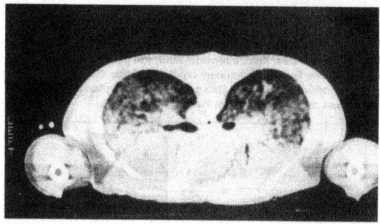

FIGURE 3-19. Computed tomographic scan of a patient with ARDS. In A, the patient is supine. In B, the patient is prone. Notice that the dependent lung is the most consolidated in both positions. (From Gattinoni L, et al. Body position changes redistribute lung computed tomographic density in patients with acute respiratory failure. Anesthesiology 1991;74:15–29.)

3-19B is a CT scan of the same patient obtained with the patient prone. Notice that most of the posterior consolidation has cleared and the posterior basal segments of the lower lobes are fairly well ventilated. If the patient were to remain prone for an hour or so, the anterior lung, which is now dependent, would become consolidated. Some of this anterior consolidation can already be seen in Figure 3-19B. How does this happen? Surely interstitial water cannot percolate directly through the lung; there is no anatomic pathway that would allow it to. And surely the posterior lung has not been instantly cleared of the edema by lymphatics. There is not enough time for

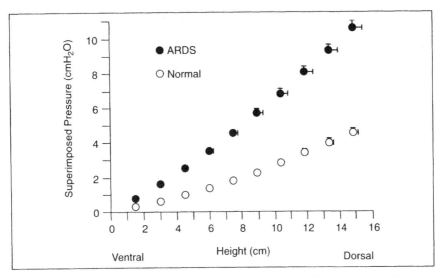

FIGURE 3-20. The amount of fluid in lung slices going from nondependent (ventral) to dependent (dorsal) as seen with CT scans. (From Pelosi P, et al. Vertical gradient of regional lung inflation in adult respiratory distress syndrome. *Am J Respir Crit Care Med.* 1994;149:8–13.)

that to have happened. We must therefore conclude that the actual amount of water in the interstitium of the lung when the patient is supine and prone is the same; it is only ventilation (and to some extent blood flow) that has changed. This leads to the conclusion that it is the weight of the upper lung pushing down on the dependent lung that causes the small airways and alveoli to collapse, leading to consolidation and transpulmonary shunting.

Conclusive proof of this theory was presented by Gattinoni using CT scans obtained from normal subjects and patient with ARDS. By calculating the Hounsfield number for each cubic centimeter of lung tissue, he showed that the amount of water in the interstitium of the ARDS lungs was roughly the same throughout, and much more than that in normal lungs. By calculating the weight of this water deeper and deeper into the dependent lung tissue, it is easy to see that the posterior aspect of the lung would be compressed, particularly if the alveoli are somewhat surfactant deficient. Add to this the weight of the abdominal viscera in the long-term supine, critically ill patient, and it is easy to see why consolidation of the posterior lower lobes is characteristic of acute respiratory failure. Some of the data from Gattinoni's paper are shown in Figure 3-20. In other studies the effect of PEEP on lung inflation has been studied by CT scanning. It is interesting to note that, once collapsed alveoli become inflated (either produced by prone positioning or by a maximal peak inflating pressure), the amount of PEEP necessary to hold these alveoli open generally corresponds to the weight of a water column that could be supported by that level of pressure. This is probably why 5 to

10 cm H_2O of PEEP is maximal in a newborn infant, whereas 20 to 30 cm H_2O is maximal in an adult. The difference is simply related to the anteroposterior diameter of the chest when the patient is supine.

The relationship of pulmonary edema to infection and fibrosis is more important than is the effect of pulmonary edema on lung function. Atelectasis may exist for weeks with no permanent effects on lung structure. However, just a few days of pulmonary edema—particularly the protein-rich, capillary leakage type of edema—sets the stage for pulmonary infection or rapidly developing fibrosis, or both. The exact mechanisms of cause and effect are not clear. Perhaps the fibrosis is a result of the primary lung injury that also led to edema, or perhaps it is the result of treatment given for the edema. In any event, humoral or airway damage to the lungs sustained over a period of days may eventuate in pulmonary destruction and fibrosis.

Management of Respiratory Failure

Our algorithm for the management of severe respiratory failure is shown in Figure 3-21. For purposes of this discussion, severe respiratory failure is defined as the need for intubation, mechanical ventilation, and supplemental inspired oxygen. Although routine ventilator patients can be managed without the placement of a pulmonary artery catheter, this device provides information essential to the effective management of severe respiratory failure and its placement is assumed for purposes of this discussion. Whenever a pulmonary artery catheter is indicated, we use a fiberoptic oximeter catheter (Oximetrix; Abbott Laboratories, Critical Care Division, Chicago) that continuously measures mixed venous saturation. We do this because most of the important steps in the management of severe respiratory failure are based on mixed venous saturation monitoring.

Although the cause of respiratory failure usually resides in the lung interstitium and parenchyma, it is important not to overlook the possibility of simple mechanical causes such as pneumothorax, hydrothorax, plugged endotracheal tubes, occluded airways, or ascites. Bronchoscopy should be carried out if there is any question of aspiration or if there is any evidence of mucous plugging or impaction in the airways. Although ventilatory management with an indwelling endotracheal tube can be maintained for days or weeks, the incidence of bacterial pneumonia associated with long-term intubation, the gas flow resistance of endotracheal tubes, and the obligatory linkage of extubation with ventilator weaning all prompt us to recommend tracheostomy rather than chronic intubation for the management of patients with severe respiratory failure. Pulmonary embolism should be considered as a cause of respiratory failure in any patient if the pulmonary artery systolic pressure is greater than 40 mm Hg.

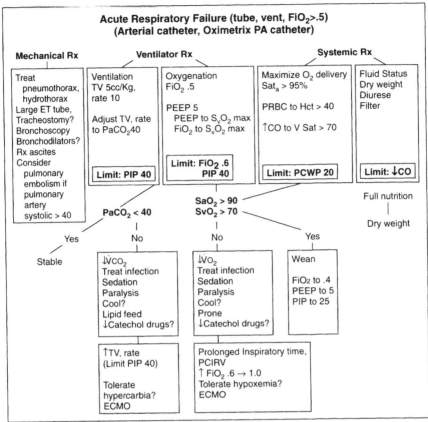

FIGURE 3-21. Respiratory failure management algorithm. (CO = cardiac output; ECMO = extracorporeal membrane oxygenation; ET = endotracheal; Hct = hematocrit; PA = pulmonary artery; PCIRV = pressure controlled inverse ratio ventilation; PCWP = pulmonary capillary wedge pressure; PE = pulmonary embolism; PEEP = positive end-expiratory pressure; PIP = peak inspiratory pressure; PRBC = packed red blood cells; SaO2 = arterial saturation; SvO2 = venous saturation; TV = tidal volume.)

Optimizing systemic oxygen delivery in relationship to oxygen requirement is the primary goal of management. Improving the oxygenation of the blood itself by improving alveolar inflation is only one of the steps in optimizing oxygen delivery. Equally or more important are treating anemia and optimizing cardiac output. Most ICU patients are anemic, and oxygen delivery is maintained by a compensatory increase in cardiac output. This is an acceptable practice because most patients have an adequate cardiac reserve to compensate for the anemia, and because of the desire to avert the potential infectious complications of blood transfusion. However, because the patient with severe respiratory failure is at risk of dying from decreased oxygen delivery (or the multiple-organ failure related thereto), the risk associated with transfusion is minor compared with the risk associated with the primary problem. This is complicated by the fact that cardiac output may be compromised in these patients, either as a result of the primary disease or of the efforts to increase oxygenation by using airway pressure. Accordingly, oxygen delivery in these patients should be optimized first by normalizing the hematocrit. Second, cardiac output should be optimal, but not necessarily maximal, to maintain delivery at a level four to five times that of consumption. In general this means avoiding those conditions that would cause cardiac output to decrease, rather than actively trying to increase cardiac output. This includes keeping the airway pressure as low as possible to maximize venous return, preventing abdominal distention, maintaining an appropriate blood volume based on a pulmonary capillary wedge pressure of approximately 15 mm Hg, and maintaining blood pressure high enough to provide coronary perfusion (mean pressure of more than 50 mm Hg), but not so high as to limit left ventricular function (mean arterial pressure of more than 90 mm Hg). If all of these steps are taken, cardiac output is usually autoregulated to maintain delivery at a level four to five times that of consumption. If myocardial contractility is inadequate, then inotropic drugs such as dopamine or dobutamine should be administered, but it should be recognized that these drugs increase both oxygen consumption and contractility. The overall benefit and titration of inotropes should be based on the mixed venous saturation measurements.

Finally, oxygen delivery can be maintained by ensuring adequate saturation of arterial blood. This can be done by supplying supplemental oxygen to the airway and by improving inflation of collapsed or poorly ventilated alveoli. The FiO_2 is increased to 50% or 60% as the initial step in the treatment of hypoxemia. Alveolar collapse is treated as outlined earlier: cleaning the airways, avoiding the administration of 100% oxygen, removing fluid from the lung or chest, and finally using PEEP to hold open those alveoli that have been opened by other measures. The optimal level of PEEP is that which maintains arterial oxygenation but does not decrease venous return or cardiac output. This optimal level is best determined by monitoring mixed venous saturation. When varying the amounts of end-expiratory pressure, the position of the patient on the pressure-volume curve should be noted and volume should be decreased if the peak airway pressure exceeds 40 cm H_2O. Another step in optimizing lung function is to take advantage of the gravitational effects on pulmonary blood flow by placing the patient prone or in a full lateral position to direct the blood flow to areas of optimal alveolar inflation. (These measures often result in the opening of closed posterior alveoli that have been compressed by the weight of fluid in the lung.)

At the same time that oxygen delivery is optimized, oxygen consumption should be decreased to normal or even below normal if necessary. Treating infection, providing adequate sedation, and establishing muscular paralysis cause oxygen consumption to decrease, and hence the need for oxygen is lessened. The degree of sedation or paralysis, as with other aspects of treatment, is based on the mixed venous saturation values. If oxygen delivery is still inadequate to meet metabolic needs despite these measures (that is, venous saturation is less than 60% to 70%), oxygen consumption can be further decreased by actively cooling the patient, but it must be borne in mind that cooling will result in coagulopathy and arrhythmias if the temperature is allowed to go below 33°C.

Optimizing CO_2 removal is usually easier than optimizing oxygen delivery. Ventilator rate and tidal volume are adjusted to achieve a normal $PaCO_2$, being careful to keep the peak airway pressure from exceeding 40 cm H_2O. If the $PaCO_2$ exceeds 45 mm Hg, the tidal volume or rate, or both, are increased until the PCO_2 is normal. CO_2 production can be minimized by sedation, paralysis, and the treatment of infection. It can be further decreased by avoiding heavy carbohydrate loads in the nutritional regimen and by cooling the patient. If the $PaCO_2$ exceeds 45 mm Hg despite these measures (and assuming tube or airway occlusion is ruled out), it is permissible to tolerate hypercapnia and achieve acid-base balance with the administration of bicarbonate or THAM (tromethamine). This is preferable to allowing extreme airway pressures of more than 40 cm H_2O to occur which would further injure the lung. Some of the other details of mechanical ventilator management are discussed in the following sections.

If oxygen delivery or CO_2 excretion continue to be inadequate despite all these measures, the patient's likelihood of survival is less than 10%. In this situation it is reasonable to consider instituting extracorporeal circulation with gas exchange (extracorporeal membrane oxygenation [ECMO]). In this procedure, catheters are placed into large vessels and venous blood is removed and oxygenated, CO_2 is removed, and the blood is returned to the arterial or venous circulation, thus providing mechanical support of pulmonary (or cardiopulmonary) function. ECMO requires systemic heparinization and a well-trained and experienced team. It is often necessary to maintain it for 1 to 4 weeks in such patients, but the current survival rate in moribund adult patients with severe respiratory failure who are supported on ECMO is over 50%.

Certain general steps must be taken in the patient with severe respiratory failure throughout the course of the illness. In particular, fluid overload should be treated with diuresis or hemofiltration until the patient is returned to dry weight. A successful outcome from the management of severe respiratory failure is correlated with overall fluid balance; fluid overload is associated with a lower survival rate. Diuresis or hemofiltration will cause the patient to become hypovolemic. As mentioned earlier, cardiac output must be supported, and the combination of diuresis and packed red blood cell transfusion is usually the best way to maintain normal blood volume in the early stages of severe respiratory failure.

Mechanical Ventilation

Mechanical ventilation should be considered when spontaneous breathing is inadequate to maintain gas exchange or when the effort needed to maintain gas exchange is exhausting the patient. Oral tracheal intubation is preferred to nasotracheal intubation, which is more uncomfortable, causes sinusitis, and requires the use of a smaller, longer tube. It is a common practice to maintain oral tracheal intubation for as long as 2 to 3 weeks, but this is probably not wise. Aside from the obvious damage to the larynx and discomfort caused by the tube, it enters the sterile airway through the grossly contaminated pharynx. Despite the best attempts at oral hygiene, the posterior pharynx harbors a slurry of virulent organisms that inevitably track down the endotracheal tube to colonize the airway, if not the alveoli. Tracheostomy is much more comfortable for the patient, confers much lower airway resistance, and most importantly, prevents contamination of the lower airway. Having been through the phase in which we favored the use of long-term intubation, we have now come to prefer early (day 1 or 2) tracheostomy for any patient with major respiratory failure. Figure 3-22 shows the potential complications related to oral tracheal intubation and tracheostomy.

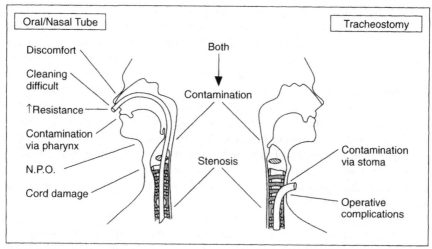

FIGURE 3-22. Potential complications related to tracheal intubation and tracheostomy for acute respiratory failure. The complications of pressure cuff injury and contamination can occur with either method of airway access, but the contamination associated with tracheostomy is much less likely and involves less virulent organisms than is the contamination through the posterior pharynx. (N.P.O. = nothing by mouth.) (From Anderson H, Bartlett RH. Respiratory care of the surgical patient. In: Burton G, Hodgkin J, Ward J, (eds). Respiratory Care, 3rd ed, 1991. Philadelphia: JB Lippincott.)

Ventilator Management

When mechanical ventilation is instituted because of coma, respiratory depression, paralysis, or weakness, or during recovery from prolonged anesthetics and operations, the lungs are normal and the intent of using mechanical ventilation is simply to provide gas exchange and keep the lungs normal until the patient is able to breathe spontaneously. In fact, mechanical ventilation is used to prevent atelectasis in patients who are recovering from major operations and might hypoventilate if extubated in the recovery room. Use of the ventilator in this basic maintenance or prophylactic mode is easy and simply requires the prevention of ventilator-induced complications. On the other extreme, mechanical ventilation is used for both life support and active treatment of the lung in severe respiratory failure. In this context, ventilator management is critical and it is possible to do more harm than good by applying damaging pressure or oxygen concentrations. Therefore the mode of mechanical ventilation chosen and the type of ventilator used depend to a large extent on the clinical application. Simple inexpensive ventilators without complicated settings and detailed monitoring capabilities are perfectly adequate for the routine or prophylactic application. Complex ventilators that are capable of monitoring and the adjustment of minute details of pressure, flow, and volume are necessary for the appropriate management of severe respiratory failure. The descriptive terms and abbreviations that have grown up with the development of mechanical ventilation are confusing and modified almost every year, but it is necessary to learn the language to use the apparatus. The terms and modes of use are best approached by examining the primary and secondary controls on the typical mechanical ventilator (Table 3-3). This initial discussion deals exclusively with volume-limited ventilation because this is the mode most widely used. Later the discussion will turn to pressure-limited ventilation, which is preferred if not required for the management of severe respiratory failure.

The primary controls, as outlined in Table 3-3, are the FiO_2, tidal volume, respiratory rate, end-expiratory pressure, and maximum inspiratory pressure safety limit. If the tidal volume is set at 10 cc/kg and the respiratory rate at 10 breaths/min, each breath will take 6 seconds (roughly 2 seconds during inspiration and 4 seconds during expiration). The minute ventilation will be 100 cc/kg/min. This is about 20% more than the normal minute ventilation, and moderate respiratory alkalosis may result, depending on the volume of CO_2 produced. For a person with normal lungs, the PEEP is set at zero, although some would say that 5 cc H_2O of PEEP is appropriate to compensate for absent glottic control, which is absent because of the endotracheal tube. Finally, the maximum inspiratory pressure safety limit is set at 40 cm H_2O because pressure above this will overdistend normal alveoli. In a patient with normal lungs, each 10-cc/kg breath requires only 10 or 15 cm H_2O of pressure generated by the ventilator. Most ventilators have alarms that are set by the operator to identify a low tidal volume, a low respiratory rate or apnea,

TABLE 3-3. Controls, Monitors, and Modes of Mechanical Ventilation

Controls	Monitors and Alarms
Primary controls	
FiO_2	—
Tidal volume (minute volume)	Tidal volume
Respiratory rate	Respiratory rate
PEEP	PEEP
Maximum inspiratory pressure	PIP
	Mean airway pressure, apnea or disconnect
Secondary controls	
Inspiratory flow rate	—
Inspiratory flow wave pattern	Inspiratory time I : E ratio
Inspiratory hold	—
Sigh rate, volume, and maximum pressure	Sigh PIP
Trigger sensitivity for assist and IMV models	—
Modes of Ventilation	
Controlled mechanical ventilation (CMV)	
Assist control (AC)	
Intermittent mandatory ventilation (IMV)	
Synchronized IMV	
Continuous positive airway pressure (CPAP)	
Pressure-controlled ventilation (PCV)	
Pressure-controlled, inverse-ratio ventilation (PC-IRV)	
Pressure support (PS)	

FiO_2 = fraction of inspired oxygen; I : E = inspiratory to expiratory; PEEP = positive end-expiratory pressure; PIP = peak inspiratory pressure.
Source: From Bartlett RH. Use of mechanical ventilation. In Holcroft J, ed. Care of the surgical patient. I: Critical care. New York: Scientific American Medicine, 1993.

a low PEEP, a high peak inspiratory pressure, and a high mean airway pressure. Using these primary controls and monitors, the ventilator is set to one of the modes identified at the bottom of Table 3-3. If the patient cannot initiate spontaneous breathing, then the ventilator is time cycled. This mode is called *controlled mechanical ventilation*. If the patient can breathe spontaneously, then the ventilator is adjusted so that a breath is delivered each time the patient initiates a breath. This is referred to as *assisted ventilation*. When there is a backup rate that initiates a mechanical breath if the patient does not initiate a spontaneous breath within a certain number of seconds, this is referred to as *assist-control ventilation*. This is the mode most widely used because the patient who controls his or her own rate of breathing will adjust that rate to achieve normocapnia, thus the need for frequent blood gas measurements is eliminated. It is possible to let patients breathe spontaneously from the ventilator without mechanical assistance, allowing them to regulate not only their own respiratory rate but also the tidal volume. This mode of spontaneous breathing is usually combined with occasional mechanically assisted large-volume breaths delivered two or three times each minute. This mode of ventilation is known as *spontaneous breathing with*

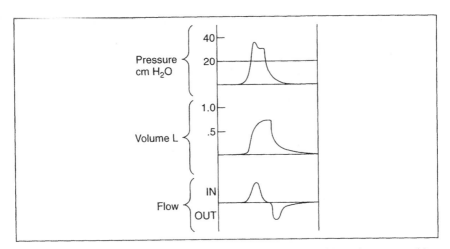

FIGURE 3-23. Pressure, flow, and volume during a typical breath generated by a time-cycled, volume-limited mechanical ventilator. (L = liter.) (From Bartlett RH. Use of mechanical ventilation. In Holcroft J, ed. Care of the surgical patient. I: Critical care. New York: Scientific American Medicine, 1993.)

intermittent mandatory ventilation (IMV). If these large-volume breaths are delivered only when a patient initiates a breath, this mode is referred to as *synchronized IMV*.

There are secondary controls on the ventilator that regulate the flow rate, flow pattern, trigger sensitivity for assisted breaths, and IMV breaths. When the ventilator is set up and the primary controls and alarms are dialed in, the pressure, volume, and flow of a single breath typically look like the tracings shown in Figure 3-23. In this example a tidal volume of 750 cc and the timed cycle or control mode of ventilation have been selected. At the beginning of the breath, gas flow begins and continues at a preset rate until the 750-cc volume has been delivered. The pressure rises rapidly in response to this volume inflation, reaching a peak of 36 cm H_2O. When the 750-cc tidal volume has been reached, gas flow stops but the expiratory valve is still held closed for 1 second because a 1-second inspiratory hold has been selected by the operator. During this inspiratory hold the pressures equilibrate, so that the pressure used for compliance calculations in this example is 30 cm H_2O. Then the expiratory valve is opened and exhalation proceeds passively. Exhalation continues until the next time-cycled breath begins, which is 6 seconds after the beginning of this breath if the respiratory rate is set at 10 breaths/min. This cycle is repeated breath after breath while the operator examines the lungs with a stethoscope, observes the respiratory effort, or lack of it, on the part of the patient, watches the pulse oximeter and the end-tidal PCO_2 monitor, and perhaps measures blood gas levels in an arterial blood sample. The FiO_2 is usually set at 50% at the initiation of mechanical ventilation, then is decreased to the level that produces an arterial saturation of between 95% and 99%, as detected with the pulse oximeter. This is done because oxygen delivery is more than ample at full saturation and FiO_2 should be maintained at the lowest level that allows full saturation to prevent displacement of nitrogen and subsequent absorption atelectasis. Using the continuous noninvasive monitors or pulse oximeter and end-tidal CO_2 monitoring, it is possible to manage patients with normal or near-normal lungs for days without measuring either arterial or venous blood gas levels.

The principles that apply to the use of the mechanical ventilator for basic maintenance or prophylaxis are exactly the same as those that apply to the management of severe respiratory failure, bearing in mind that the levels of pressure and oxygen necessary to achieve normal blood gas levels might be very damaging to the lung. Under these circumstances it is safer to accept moderate hypoxemia and hypercapnia than to strive for total normalization of the blood gas levels. Suppose the settings just outlined, consisting of an FiO_2 of 50%, tidal volume of 10 cc/kg, and respiratory rate of 10 breaths/min, are initiated in a patient with severe respiratory failure but the resulting arterial saturation is only 85% and the end-tidal and/or arterial P_{CO_2}, is 55 mm Hg. How should the ventilator settings be modified? First of all, it is important to realize that adjustments aimed at normalizing oxygenation are quite different from the adjustments aimed at normalizing P_{CO_2}. CO_2 clearance is achieved by increasing alveolar ventilation through the regulation of the respiratory rate and tidal volume, taking care not to exceed a peak inspiratory pressure of 40 cm H_2O. Oxygenation is facilitated by increasing the peak inspiratory pressure to achieve inflation (but not to more than 40 cm H_2O) and increasing PEEP to hold inflation. These approaches may be mutually exclusive. For example, increasing PEEP while limiting the peak inspiratory pressure will result in a smaller tidal volume. If this is the case, it is better to err on the side of adequate oxygenation and allow hypercapnia.

For the past 25 years, volume-limited ventilation has been the preferred mode of ventilation in adult ICUs. Large tidal volumes were the rule regardless of the inflating pressure required to squeeze the volume in. In the past few years it has been widely recognized that this was a mistake. The high pressures overinflated the most normal alveoli in the lungs, resulting in capillary stretching, capillary leakage, more pulmonary edema, alveolar rupture, and often pleural rupture leading to pneumothorax. This barotrauma can occur with only a few breaths at high pressure, forcing a large tidal volume into partially inflated lungs. (The trauma is actually volutrauma resulting in overdistention rather than pressure-induced barotrauma.) For years this volutrauma was attributed to PEEP, because these patients were treated with PEEP at fixed tidal volumes at the highest peak inspiratory pressure. It is now clear that the injury is caused by a high peak inspiratory pressure and overdistention rather than a high mean or end-expiratory pressure. Now, in one of the most rapid turnarounds in worldwide intensive care management, the peak inspiratory pressure is limited to 40 cm H_2O. Some would say that even 40 cm H_2O is too high, favoring pressures closer to 30 cm H_2O. In any event, it is generally recognized that overdistention must be avoided and, if hypercapnia or hypoxemia results, that that is safer than the use of higher pressures or volumes. This practice has reminded us of some elementary facts regarding tolerance to hypercapnia and hypoxia. Respiratory acidosis causes very few side effects. Patients can do very well with a PaCO$_2$ of 80 mm Hg and a pH of 7.1 lasting for hours or days. We have all cared for patients with asthma or chronic obstructive pulmonary disease who do very well despite PCO$_2$s in the 60s. Hypoxemia is also well tolerated as long as the systemic oxygen delivery is adequate. Using the principles discussed earlier in this chapter, it can be seen that it is much safer to transfuse red blood cells, use low doses of inotropic drugs, and decrease the volume of oxygen consumed by inducing paralysis and hypothermia than it is to raise the FiO$_2$ to more than 60%. In the early days of cardiac surgery we all cared for perfectly functional children who lived for many years breathing air with PaO$_2$ in the 30s.

When the lung recovers from acute respiratory failure (or when the postoperative patient is fully alert and awake), it is time to think about weaning him or her from mechanical ventilation to resume spontaneous breathing. Some simple measurements of lung function and pulmonary mechanics can assure us that the patient is ready for extubation and spontaneous breathing. The SaO$_2$ should be greater than 90% at an FiO$_2$ of 0.4 or less. The patient should be able to generate an inspiratory force exceeding 20 cm H$_2$O and a spontaneous vital capacity at least twice the tidal volume. If an end-tidal PCO$_2$ monitor is used, the end-tidal CO$_2$ pressure should be less than 40 mm Hg. These weaning parameters are summarized in Table 3-4. When the patient meets these parameters he or she is disconnected from the ventilator (or the ventilator is adjusted to provide a constant gas flow at no significant inflating pressure) and is encouraged to breathe regularly and deeply. The respiratory rate and the pulse rate are monitored, the latter to provide a rough estimate of the work of breathing, because if the patient has to exert a lot of energy to sustain breathing, the pulse rate rises steadily. If the patient is able to breathe deeply and spontaneously at a rate of less than 20 breaths/min and a pulse rate of less than 90 beats/min, he or she is extubated. It is always easier to breathe through the normal airway than through the endotracheal tube, so the respiratory rate and pulse rate will be even lower after extubation. If the respiratory rate is more than 30 breaths/min or the pulse rate is more than

TABLE 3-4. Weaning Parameters

Parameter	Result	
Inspiratory force	> 20 cm H$_2$O	spontaneous breathing
Tidal volume	5 cc/kg	
Vital capacity	10 cc/kg	
Minute ventilation	1 L/10 kg/min	on ventilator
SaO$_2$ (on FiO$_2$ < 4, PEEP < 5)	>95%	

FiO$_2$ = fraction of inspired oxygen; PEEP = positive end-expiratory pressure; SaO$_2$ = arterial oxygen saturation.

84 Critical Care Physiology

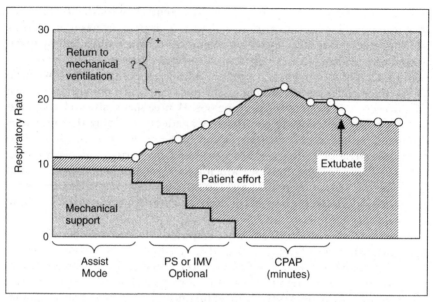

FIGURE 3-24. After a brief period of spontaneous breathing or pressure support (*PS*), the patient is extubated if the respiratory rate is less than 20 breaths/min. (CPAP = continuous positive airway pressure; IMV = intermittent mandatory ventilation.)

100 beats/min, the patient will probably not tolerate extubation and should be returned to mechanical ventilation until the problem is identified and eradicated. If the pulse and respiration are in the intermediate zone, the decision whether to extubate or not is based on the degree of oxygenation and CO_2 clearance as shown by pulse oximetry and end-tidal measurement or by the arterial blood gas levels (Figure 3-24).

Some patients may have adequate or borderline weaning parameters but fail spontaneous breathing trials or require intubation after extubation. Our protocol for dealing with these difficult-to-wean patients is shown in Figure 3-25. If a tracheostomy has not already been done, it is the first and often most important step in managing the patient who is difficult to wean from the ventilator. Aside from the comfort and bacteriologic benefits of a tracheostomy mentioned earlier, in a difficult-to-wean patient the tracheostomy decreases the dead space or rebreathing space by approximately 50 cc. It also considerably decreases the airway resistance because the short tracheostomy tube has much less resistance than the longer endotracheal tube. Even more important than these principles of physics are the practical principles relative to the risk of extubation. The designation "difficult ventilator weaning" often means that the patient is being kept on a ventilator simply because, if thick secretions or hypoventilation develops hours or days after extubation, a respiratory disaster might occur before the patient could be electively or

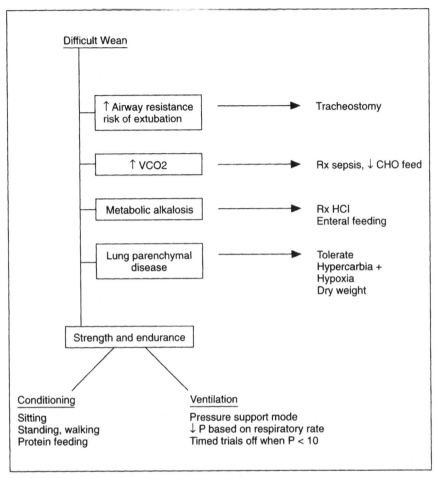

FIGURE 3-25. Protocol for management of patients who are difficult to wean from mechanical ventilation. (CHO = carbohydrate; P = pressure; Rx = treatment; VCO_2 = CO_2 production.)

urgently reintubated. So the patient remains on the ventilator because of the nervousness of the care team responsible. All this concern is eliminated by a tracheostomy. In addition, it is much easier to get the patient out of bed, sitting in a chair, standing, and walking by the bedside. Trials of spontaneous breathing through the tracheostomy tube are simple and carry no risks, whereas trials of spontaneous breathing through an endotracheal tube are exhausting for the patient and unsettling for the nursing staff. For all these reasons, difficult-to-wean patients often are completely off the ventilator within a day or two after a tracheostomy has been done. The second step in managing the difficult-to-wean patient is to measure the respiratory quotient and assure that CO_2 production is kept to a minimum. Because ventilator weaning is in essence a breathing exercise, and because the reason for breathing is CO_2 elimination, the amount of breathing that is necessary is determined by the rate of CO_2 production. Increased metabolic activity such as that caused by sepsis or unnecessary muscular effort should be minimized. Enteral and parenteral feeding should be adjusted so that the predominant substrate is fat and the total calories are slightly less than the resting energy expenditure. This will drive the respiratory quotient down to 0.7 or 0.8, thereby proportionately decreasing the need for alveolar ventilation. Metabolic alkalosis is the most common abnormality of acid-base balance in the ICU and is caused by chronic gastric acid removal, the effects of diuretics, and the presence of lactate or acetate in intravenous fluids. If the patient has metabolic alkalosis and is difficult to wean from the ventilator, the alkalosis should be treated with intravenous infusions of 0.1 normal hydrochloric acid until a P_{CO_2} of 40 mm Hg is associated with a pH of 7.4.

After these three practical steps are taken, it should be determined whether ventilator weaning might be limited by the existence of lung parenchymal disease, particularly residual lung injury manifested as honeycombing (alveolar gas space without blood supply), and interstitial fibrosis. These conditions often take months to resolve, and ultimately the patient may have to be weaned from the ventilator with moderate hypercapnia and hypoxia. Pulmonary edema should be treated, if present, to maintain the patient at dry weight. Often elderly patients with cardiac disease must be carefully balanced between pulmonary edema and congestive heart failure, requiring a left atrial pressure of 20 cm H_2O for adequate cardiac function but suffering pulmonary edema at a pressure of 22 or 23 cm H_2O. In these patients it is necessary to have a pulmonary artery catheter in place to facilitate ventilator weaning. However, in most patients who are difficult to wean, one of the important steps is to remove central pulmonary artery catheters, central venous catheters, and arterial catheters; this has three benefits. First, the patient is much more mobile and can stand or sit at the bedside without the risk of dislodging catheters. Second, all of the monitoring is then focused on pulse oximetry and end-tidal CO_2 pressure measurements, thus decreasing the temptation to focus on minor ventilator changes. Third, the patient who is free of monitoring catheters is no longer considered critically ill but rather graduated to rehab status. This simple change in the perception of the patient's condition on the part of the patient, the family, and the care team results in a different approach to management and some evidence that the formerly critically ill patient is now well on the road to recovery.

Once all of these preliminary steps in preparation for ventilator weaning are accomplished, all that remains is strength and endurance training. Although sitting up in bed or at the bedside facilitates breathing, nothing works as well or as quickly as standing. In addition to the postural benefits of standing (see Figure 3-4), there is something about using the postural support muscles that enhances the strength and endurance of the respiratory muscles. Standing in this context does not mean a few seconds of pivoting from the bed to the bedside chair but bearing all the weight on the feet for an hour or two at a time. For the elderly or frail patient to stand who has just spent 2 or 3 weeks on bed rest, often pharmacologically paralyzed, requires the use of a circle bed with a footboard and gradually progressive tilting to the full upright position. *Gradual* in this context does not mean over the course of a week or two, but an hour spent at 50 degrees, then at 75 degrees, then at 80 degrees, and then fully upright.

One of the least important details of strength and endurance testing is the one that inevitably receives the most attention, namely management of the ventilator itself. Pressure-limited rather than volume-limited ventilation should be used, and the pressure support mode available in newer ventilators is preferred. When weaning difficult-to-wean patients, the pressure limit is progressively decreased based on the pressure needed to maintain the patient's spontaneous respiratory rate at around 20 to 30 breaths/minute. These adjustments in ventilator pressure, the backup IMV rate, and the like, should be made by the nursing and respiratory staff based on the respiratory rate, end-tidal CO_2 pressure, and pulse oximetry data without the measurement of blood gas levels and without physician intervention or written orders every time the ventilator is changed. When the pressure limit is down to about 10 cm H_2O, the patient is ready for spontaneous breathing trials with no supplemental assistance from the ventilator. These trials should be done with the patient sitting or standing and should progress rapidly from a few minutes to several hours, then to daytime breathing, then to freedom from the ventilator altogether. When a patient is breathing spontaneously through a tracheostomy (or endotracheal) tube, the balloon cuff should be deflated so that, if the tube becomes occluded with a mucous plug, the patient can still breathe around the tube while getting the attention of the nursing staff. This leads to the dilemma of how to deal with airway secretions with the tube in place. The patient may be strong enough to be weaned off the ventilator but still appears to need ICU care because of the requirement for frequent suctioning. The presence of an artificial airway, particularly when the cuff is deflated and minor episodes of aspiration occur frequently, causes mucus to accumulate in the airway, which in turn requires frequent suctioning. Usually the best way to deal with this problem is to simply remove the tracheostomy tube altogether. It is possible to suction airway secretions through the stoma for a few days after the tube has been removed, and this simple step often solves the problem.

Learning to Manage Mechanical Ventilators

Although the principles of mechanical ventilation are well standardized, the actual devices appear to be quite different. Each ICU has a standard ventilator that is used for most patients, with other ventilators available for special purposes or to meet personal preferences. In most hospitals in the United

States, ventilators are maintained and managed by respiratory therapists. Indeed, in most U.S. hospitals, touching the controls of a mechanical ventilator has become the exclusive domain of the respiratory therapists (elsewhere in the world ventilators are managed by nurses and physicians). Whatever the policy in a given ICU, the physician charged with managing the patient's care must be familiar with all aspects of the mechanical ventilator being used in that particular unit. Respiratory therapy is a wonderful resource, and the attending physician should take full advantage of the opportunity to learn from the respiratory therapists all the major and minor details of each ventilator in the unit. The best way to do this is to put yourself on the ventilator using a noseclip and a mouthpiece, then run the ventilator through settings until you have a thorough understanding of how that particular ventilator can be adjusted and how it feels to the patient. The best mouthpiece is an endotracheal tube with the balloon inflated and held inside the mouth. This gives you the feeling the patient has when relying on this long, narrow airway for breathing. Protocol for self-instruction on the use of a mechanical ventilator is shown in Table 3-5. To avoid suffocation, panic, and embarrassment, it is best to start with a rubber bag (or better yet an adjustable mechanical test lung available from your respiratory therapy department) to become familiar with the initial settings, then go through all the modes of ventilation with yourself as the test subject. If it is available, use a continuous pulmonary mechanics monitor to measure your progress.

TABLE 3-5. Self-instruction Routine for Mechanical Ventilator Training

1. Set FiO_2, V_T, rate, PEEP and PIP.
2. Set mode: CMV.
3. Set ranges for alarms: V_T, rate, PIP, and PEEP.
4. Attach test lung (rubber bag) and ventilate
5. Measure V_T, rate, minute volume, PIP, PEEP, and effective compliance.
6. Limit the bag to simulate poor compliance. Readjust ventilator and repeat measurements.
7. Set primary controls to ventilate yourself: rate = 16 breaths/min.
8. With a mouthpiece and a noseclip in place, ventilate yourself. Relax until you are on controlled ventilation. Then adjust V_T (5–20 mL/kg) and PEEP (0–10 cm H_2O) to get the feel and observe the measurements. Try the sigh mode.
9. At baseline settings, resist inspiration, cough, and try to hyperventilate. How does it feel? Do the monitors and alarms work?
10. At baseline settings, turn to the AC mode: rate = 0 breaths/min. Adjust the sensitivity from low to high.
11. In the AC mode, adjust the inspiratory flow rate and pattern. Which I:E ratio feels comfortable?
12. Reset mode to IMV, then CPAP. How much work does it take to initiate a breath?
13. Repeat steps 10 to 12, but using an endotracheal tube in your mouth instead of a mouthpiece. What are the effects of the added resistance?

CMV = controlled mechanical ventilation; CPAP = continuous positive airway pressure; FiO_2 = fraction of inspired oxygen; I:E = inspiratory to expiratory; PEEP = positive end-expiratory pressure; PIP = peak inspiratory pressure; V_T = tidal volume.

Mechanical Ventilation in Severe Respiratory Failure

As we have frequently emphasized in this chapter, the management of the patient with severe respiratory failure includes many factors, the least important of which is the settings on the mechanical ventilator. Improper management of the ventilator will worsen rather than ameliorate the respiratory failure. On the other hand, there are occasions when ventilator adjustments actually bring about an improvement in lung inflation and function. Simply summarized, the safe limits of mechanical ventilation are an FiO_2 of 50%, peak inspiratory pressure of 30 cm H_2O, PEEP of 10 cm H_2O, and respiratory rate of 20 breaths/min. If these limits were arbitrarily imposed, deaths from acute respiratory failure in ICUs would decrease rather than increase. The mortality associated with exceeding these settings is 40%. (More accurately, the mortality associated with respiratory failure that the physician perceives as severe enough to require exceeding these settings is 40%.) Nonetheless, there are some situations in which ventilator adjustments in the high range are necessary and result in recovery.

The principles relating to the management of pulmonary mechanics in patients with severe respiratory failure are summarized in Figure 3-26. Simple volume-limited ventilation, as already discussed and demonstrated in Figure 3-24, is shown in this figure as the first example and identified as *IMV* or *CMV* (controlled volume ventilation). In Figure 3-26 the event that begins the mechanical breath cycle is identified by a triangle. After this initiating event the ventilator delivers gas into the patient until a limit (identified by a black triangle in Figure 3-26) is reached. Inspiratory gas flow then stops and the expiratory valve is held closed if a plateau pressure has been selected. After this the expiratory valve opens and passive exhalation ensues until the mechanical breathing cycle begins again. Routine ventilation can be done with either a volume or pressure limit, but management of the patient with severe respiratory failure is best done with pressure-limited ventilation, identified as *PCV* in Figure 3-26. Pressure-limited ventilation is preferred because one of the major problems is always lung consolidation. In addition to maintaining adequate gas exchange, one of the goals of mechanical ventilation is to recruit the collapsed alveoli in the consolidated areas while preventing overdistention of the normal alveoli. This recruitment is done during the inflation phase of mechanical ventilation, then the recruited alveoli are held open by PEEP, awaiting more recruitment with the next breath. When alveoli are recruited, the FRC becomes larger and the compliance is therefore lower. When pressure-limited ventilation is used, this breath-to-breath improvement in compliance results in a breath-to-breath increase in the tidal volume that recruits evermore alveoli. (In the volume-limited mode the peak inspiratory pressure declines as compliance improves, thereby any advantage in the recruitment of more alveoli is lost.) Because alveoli are recruited while at peak inspiratory pressure, there is significant advantage to making this time as long as is safe and tolerable. This is done by applying plateau pressure.

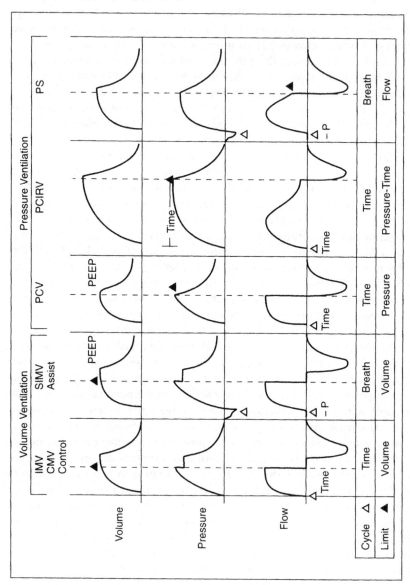

FIGURE 3-26

3. Respiratory Physiology and Pathophysiology

When plateau pressure is used in conjunction with pressure-limited ventilation, inspiratory flow continues (rather than the expiratory valve simply being capped, as occurs in volume-limited ventilation). The plateau is set by determining the total inspiratory time that the peak inspiratory pressure is applied, rather than the time that the expiratory valve is closed after full inflation. Used in this fashion to best advantage, the inspiratory time may be equal to, or even considerably longer than, the expiratory time, resulting in a reversal of the usual inspiratory-to-expiratory ratio. This application of pressure-limited ventilation has been called *pressure-controlled, inverse-ratio ventilation* or PCIRV. This mode of ventilation is very effective in recruiting the collapsed alveoli associated with major respiratory failure. However, it runs the risk of causing a high mean intrathoracic pressure that may inhibit venous return, and is unnatural and uncomfortable for the patient, so that heavy sedation or paralysis is usually required. Try it on yourself, but limit your respiratory rate to 5 or 6 breaths/min, otherwise respiratory alkalosis will rapidly occur.

When a consolidated lung has been expanded and it is possible to decrease the minute ventilation and think about weaning, the pressure limit is gradually decreased as long as adequate inflation and minute ventilation are sustained. The major problem with pressure-limited ventilation is that atelectasis or airway mucous plugs that decrease compliance will immediately decrease the volume of any pressure-limited breath, so careful attention must be given to tidal volume monitoring (just as pressure must be monitored during volume-limited ventilation). One way of dealing with this problem is to use a variation of pressure-limited ventilation in which the breathing cycle is initiated by the patient and the prescribed pressure limit is reached, but inspiration is limited by gas flow rather than by either pressure or volume. This results in a very natural-feeling breath and is ideal for weaning patients from mechanical ventilation. This mode of ventilator control is commonly called *pressure support*. Some ventilators include a mode in which the problem of atelectasis with decreasing pressure-limited breaths is addressed by continuing the flow, if necessary, until a prescribed volume is reached. This variation is called *volume-assured pressure support* (VAPS).

FIGURE 3-26. Patterns of mechanical ventilation. All ventilators generate gas flow that starts (cycle, control–control: △) based on a timer or is triggered by patient inhalation ($-P$). Gas flow stops (limit: ▲) when a preset volume, pressure, or flow is reached. Volume-limited ventilation should always be used with an inspiratory hold or plateau. Two examples show the effect of PEEP. (CMV = controlled mechanical ventilation; IMV = intermittent mandatory ventilation; PCIRV = pressure-controlled inverse ratio ventilation; PCV = pressure-controlled ventilation; PS = pressure support; SIMV = synchronized intermittent mandatory ventilation.) (From Bartlett RH. Use of mechanical ventilation. In: Holcroft J, ed. Care of the surgical patient. I: Critical care. New York: Scientific American Medicine, 1993.)

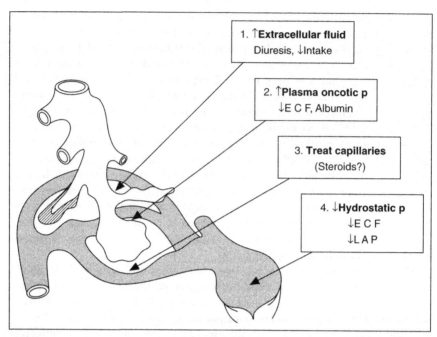

FIGURE 3-27. Treatment of increased lung water. (E C F = extracellular fluid; L A P = left atrial pressure; P = pressure.) (From: Bartlett RH. Respiratory care of surgical patient. Surgical Clin North Am Vol. 62, No. 1, 1980.)

Treatment of the Interstitial Space

Most patients with severe respiratory failure have abnormally permeable pulmonary capillaries secondary to local inflammation and infection (in the case of pneumonia) or secondary to systemic factors (such as endotoxemia and intravascular coagulation). This increased permeability leads to the transudation of plasma into the pulmonary interstitium. It is cleared by pulmonary lymphatics, but if the filtration rate exceeds the capability of lymphatics to clear the plasma, edema will result (see Figure 3-17). Edema fluid migrates within the lung to the loose areolar tissue surrounding pulmonary arterioles and small bronchi, leading to an increase in pulmonary vascular resistance and decreased ventilation in the edematous area. Changes in lung function do not occur until the lung water content is more than twice normal; therefore the patient with interstitial edema who is symptomatic has a major disturbance of transcapillary kinetics. Treatment of the edema has two important goals (Figure 3-27). The first is to improve oxygenation if it is impaired, and the second is to minimize fibrosis and bacterial infection, which often accompany the pulmonary edema stemming from capillary injury. (Fibrosis and infection are unusual after hydrostatic edema.) The treatment of interstitial edema consists of maintaining the hydrostatic pressure as low as is compatible with adequate cardiac output

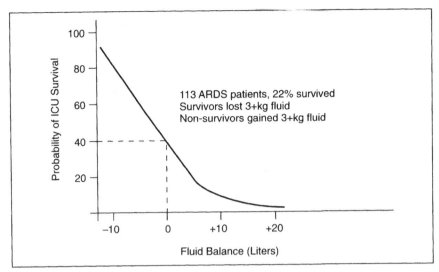

FIGURE 3-28. Outcome related to fluid balance on day 4 in ARDS patients. (Data from: Simmons RS, et al. Fluid balance in the adult respiratory distress syndrome. Am Rev Respir Dis 1987;135:924-9.)

and raising the oncotic pressure selectively in the vascular space. These measures, combined with fluid restriction and diuresis, will reduce the pulmonary edema. Regulating the hydrostatic pressure and cardiac output requires the use of a pulmonary artery catheter and frequent determinations of cardiac output. Simmons and colleagues found that survival in 113 patients with ARDS correlated with a negative fluid balance (Figure 3-28). Twenty-two percent of their patients survived. Survivors showed weight loss and a negative fluid balance (3-kg loss by day 5); nonsurvivors showed weight gain and a positive fluid balance (3-kg gain by day 5).

Because it is desirable to maintain the filling pressure of the left ventricle as low as possible while maintaining a good cardiac output, inotropic drugs are helpful in improving left ventricular contractility. Dobutamine or dopamine should be used and titrated to optimize venous saturation. A Frank-Starling curve can be constructed and the optimal combination of filling pressure and dosage of inotropic drug determined.

Simple extracellular fluid overload may contribute to the development of interstitial edema in the lung. For example, in some centers it is common practice to infuse 5 to 10 liters of saline solution along with blood replacement in trauma patients. This is done as an attempt to replace presumed losses into the "third" extracellular space. (The plasma volume and the interstitial fluid are the normal extracellular spaces; the pathophysiologic "third" space is the transient edema in the area of operation or injury.) This third space will expand as long as salt water is poured into the patient, and the difference between what is required and what is actually given is often

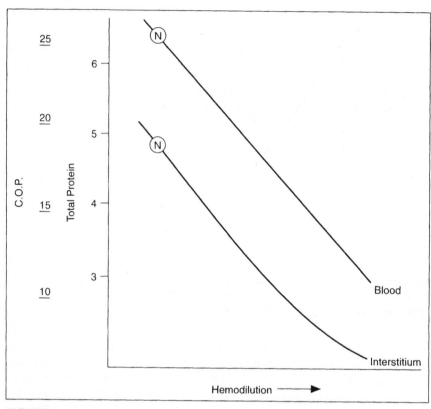

FIGURE 3-29. Relationship between plasma oncotic pressure (*C.O.P.* in mm Hg) and plasma protein level (g/dL). (Ⓝ = normal.)

measured in liters. One might wonder why gross pulmonary edema does not result each time this type of fluid overload occurs. The reason is that the interstitial proteins, as well as the plasma proteins, are equally diluted with colloid-free electrolyte solution, thus maintaining the oncotic gradient across the pulmonary capillary bed (Figure 3-29). This was demonstrated nicely by Demling and associates, who resuscitated animals from hemorrhage through the administration of different solutions and measured the composition of the pulmonary lymph. They found that the plasma and lymph protein concentrations decreased at a rate commensurate with the rate of progressive hemodilution, maintaining the oncotic gradient across the pulmonary capillary at plasma albumin levels as low as 1.3 g/dL. The fact that most patients tolerate iatrogenic edema does not mean that this is a good practice. If sepsis occurs in an edematous patient, the increased capillary permeability may lead to pulmonary, myocardial, or brain dysfunction.

As mentioned earlier, pulmonary edema does not result in dysfunction until the lung water content is more than twice normal, but once alveolar flooding begins, small increments of edema cause major dysfunction. For the same reason, removal of a small amount of edematous fluid from the lung may result in major improvement.

The first step in decreasing pulmonary edema is to decrease the pulmonary capillary hydrostatic pressure to as low a level as is compatible with an adequate cardiac output.

This is done by diuresis and fluid restriction. As the patient falls behind in blood volume, signs of hypovolemia may appear. Blood volume is then replenished with a fluid that stays in the vascular space. Packed red blood cells are ideal for this purpose. When the hematocrit is normal, concentrated salt-poor albumin should be used. This hyperoncotic fluid replenishes the blood volume by attracting interstitial fluid from throughout the body into the vascular space and supplementing diuresis. This technique is useful even in the septic patient who may have increased capillary permeability and may rapidly lose albumin from the vascular space. Even if albumin "leaks out" at a rate three or four times normal, the short-term effects of expanding blood volume and decreasing edema will appear. Experience with the infusion of albumin solutions into patients who are already hypervolemic has led to the mistaken impression that the use of concentrated albumin in the *hypo*volemic patient may cause problems. On the contrary, it is an efficient way to reexpand blood volume. The use of concentrated globulins would be better yet, but such a preparation is not available. Although furosemide is customarily used as the diuretic of choice, mannitol should be considered. This drug produces osmotic diuresis as well as a transient plasma hyperosmolarity, thus "pulling" fluid into the vascular space.

All the principles of physiology, physics, and common sense discussed in this chapter come together in the management algorithm and the respiratory care axioms (Table 3-6).

TABLE 3-6. Respiratory Failure Axioms

1. Breathing and ventilation is for CO_2 removal; inflation is for oxygenation.
2. Normalize O_2 delivery, not just PaO_2.
3. Oxygenation management (FiO_2, position, suction, PEEP, and inotropes) is based on SvO_2.
4. In apnea, hypoxemia is fatal in minutes. Hypercapnia alone is never fatal.
5. Increasing FiO_2 decreases the alveolar nitrogen concentration and causes atelectasis.
6. Mechanical ventilation does more harm than good at high PIP and high FiO_2.
7. Never exceed EIP (plateau) of more than 40 cm H_2O. Hypercapnia is safer than EIP of more than 40 cm H_2O.
8. Ventilation management (rate, pressure, and volume) is based on the $PaCO_2$ or end-tidal CO_2 pressure.
9. Achieve and maintain dry weight.
10. Do not confuse pulmonary capillary wedge pressure with hydration status.

FiO_2 = fraction of inspired oxygen; PaO_2 = arterial oxygen pressure; EIP = end inspiratory pressure; SvO_2 = venous oxygen saturation.

Monographs and Reviews

Arensman R, Cornish D, eds. Extracorporeal life support. Boston, Oxford: Blackwell, 1993.
   This multi-authored monograph summarizes the research and clinical experience with extracorporeal life support for the treatment of cardiac and respiratory failure.

Bartels H, ed. Methods in pulmonary physiology. New York, London: Hafner, 1963.
   This classic monograph describes in great detail the instrumentation and methods used in respiratory physiology. It is an invaluable reference for a critical care physician.

Bartlett RH. Post traumatic pulmonary insufficiency. In: Cooper P, Nyhus L, eds. Surgery Annual, 1971. New York: Appleton-Century-Crofts, 1971.
   This chapter has concise descriptions of normal and abnormal respiratory physiology in the setting of critical illness. Several figures from this chapter are included in this text.

Bartlett RH, ed. Respiratory care of the surgical patient. Surg Clin North Am Vol. 62, No. 6, 1980.
   This multiauthored monograph includes several practical reviews of respiratory physiology and monitoring. Several figures and concepts from the chapter on pulmonary pathophysiology in surgical patients from this monograph are included or described in this text.

Bartlett RH. Use of mechanical ventilation. In: Holcroft J, ed. Care of the surgical patient. 1: Critical care. New York: Scientific American Medicine, 1993.
   Several concepts and figures used in this text are taken from this chapter.

Gattinoni L, Bombino M, Pelosi P, et al. Lung structure and function in different stages of severe adult respiratory distress syndrome. JAMA 1994;271:1772–9.
   A summary of a series of landmark studies conducted by the Gattinoni group.

Nunn JF, ed. Applied respiratory physiology. London: Butterworths, 1969.
   The sections on mechanical ventilation are particularly good.

Shanley CJ, Bartlett RH. The management of acute respiratory failure. Current Opin Gen Surg 1994;7–16.
   The University of Michigan algorithm for the management of severe respiratory failure is described in this chapter.

West JB. Respiratory physiology; Respiratory pathophysiology; Ventilation/blood flow and gas exchange. London: Blackwell, 1970.
   These classic monographs written by the dean of modern pulmonary physiologists are written for medical students but constitute the best, most concise standard reference in respiratory physiology.

Selected Reports

Albert RK, Leasa D, Sanderson M, et al. Prone positioning improves arterial oxygenation and reduces shunt in oleic acid induced acute lung injury. Am Rev Respir Dis 1987;135:628–33.
   This animal study demonstrated that decreased shunting occurs in the prone position. Several clinical studies, such as the one described in the Gattinoni paper, have also assessed the merits of the prone position.

3. Respiratory Physiology and Pathophysiology 97

Artigas A, Carlet J, LeGall JR, et al. Clinical presentation prognostic factors and outcome of ARDS in the European collaborative study, 1985–1987. A preliminary report. In: Zapol WM, Lamaire F, eds. Adult respiratory distress syndrome. New York: Dekker, 1991.
This is the first report of the European collaborative (Euroxy) study identifying the epidemiology of ARDS in Europe.

Ashbaugh DG, Bigelow DB, Petty TL, Levine BE. Acute respiratory distress in adults. Lancet 1967;2:319–23.
Description of acute respiratory failure in which the term adult respiratory distress syndrome was first used.

Bartlett RH, Morris AH, Fairley HB, et al. A prospective study of acute hypoxic respiratory failure. Chest 1986;89:684–89.
A nine-center study of the epidemiology and natural history of acute respiratory failure in adults. One of the first studies to examine the progressive mortality associated with multiple-organ failure.

Bernard GR, Artigas A, Brigham KL, et al. The American-European consensus conference on ARDS. Definitions, mechanisms, relative outcomes, and clinical trial coordination. Am J Respir Crit Care Med 1994;149:818–24.
This is the report of a consensus conference on ARDS held in 1992 that was very helpful in providing definitions, describing epidemiology, and planning future studies. The same report was published in the Journal of Critical Care *in March 1994.*

Bone RC, Maunder R, Slotman G, Silverman H, Hyers TM, Kerstein MD, Ursprung JJ. An early test of survival in patients with the adult respiratory distress syndrome. The PaO_2/FiO_2 ratio and its differential response to conventional therapy. Chest 1989;96:849–51.
A series review in which the PaO_2/FiO_2 ratio is introduced.

Gattinoni L, D'Andrea L, Pelosi P, Vitale G, Pesenti A, Fumagalli R. Regional effects and mechanism of positive end-expiratory pressure in early adult respiratory distress syndrome. JAMA 1993;269:2122–27.
PEEP acts by lifting up the weight of wet lung that would otherwise cause small airways and alveoli to collapse.

Gattinoni L, Pelosi P, Vitale G, Pesenti A, D'Andrea L, Masheroni D. Body position changes redistribute lung computed tomographic density in patients with acute respiratory failure. Anesthesiology 1991;74:15–29.
The first anatomic (CT) description of the effect of the prone position on lung inflation.

Gattinoni L, Pesenti A, Avalli L., Rossi F, Bombino M. Pressure-volume curve of total respiratory system in acute respiratory failure: a computed tomographic study. Am Rev Respir Dis 1987;136:730–6.
Correlation of the anatomic features with the pulmonary mechanics of ARDS.

Hechtman HB, Weisel RD, Vito L, et al. The independence of pulmonary shunting and pulmonary edema. Surgery 1973;74:300–6.
This paper very nicely demonstrates the difference in the pathophysiologic features of pulmonary edema and a transpulmonary shunt. A large shunt can exist without edema (atelectasis), and edema can exist without a shunt if the lungs are well ventilated.

Hernandez LA, Peevy KJ, Moise AA, Parker JC. Chest wall restriction limits high airway pressure-induced lung injury in young rabbits. J Appl Physiol 1989; 66:2364–8.

This study demonstrates that overdistention (not pressure per se) is the cause of the high-pressure alveolar change.

Hickling KG, Henderson SJ, Jackson R. Low mortality associated with low volume pressure limited ventilation with permissive hypercapnia in severe adult respiratory distress syndrome. Intensive Care Med 1990;16:372–7.

The term permissive hypercapnia is introduced in this paper emphasizing peak-pressure limits.

Hickling KG, Walsh J, Henderson S, Jackson R. Low mortality rate in ARDS using low volume, pressure-limited ventilation with permissive hypercapnia: a prospective study. Crit Care Med 1994;22:1568–78.

Survival is improved as the result of pressure limitation in patients with ARDS, compared with the survival in historical controls and patients in contemporary published series.

Hurst JM, Branson RD, Davis JK, Barrette RR, Adams KS. Comparison of conventional ventilation and high frequency jet ventilation. Ann Surg 1990;211:486–91.

High-frequency ventilation can clear CO_2 but offers no advantages.

Kolobow TA, Moretti MP, Fumagali R. Severe impairment of lung function induced by high peak airway pressure during mechanical ventilation: an experimental study. Am Rev Respir Dis 1987;135:312–5.

Lung injury occurred in normal sheep ventilated at 50 cm H_2O for 1 day. Some of the injury may be due to tissue alkalosis.

Lamm WJE, Graham MM, Albert RK. Mechanism by which the prone position improves oxygenation in acute lung injury. Am J Respir Crit Care Med 1994; 150:184–93.

Prone positioning redistributes blood flow to the anterior aspect of the lung and improves inflation of the posterior aspect.

Manthous CA, Schmidt GA. Inverse ratio ventilation in ARDS. Improved oxygenation without auto PEEP. Chest 1993;103:953–4.

A description of the physiologic response to pressure-controlled, inverse-ratio ventilation.

Morel D, Dargent F, Bachman M, et al. Pulmonary extraction of serotonin and propanolol in patients with ARDS. Am Rev Respir Dis 1985;132:479–84.

The Geneva scoring system of ARDS was introduced in this experimental study.

Mitchell JP, Schuller D, Calandrino FS, Schuster DP. Improved outcome based on fluid management in critically ill patients requiring pulmonary artery catheterization. Am Rev Respir Dis 1992;145:990–8.

ARDS patients had a better result when managed by algorithms intended to lower the pulmonary artery pressure and induce diuresis.

Morris A, Wallace CJ, Menlove R et al. A randomized clinical trial of pressure-controlled inverse ratio ventilation and extracorporeal CO_2 removal for adult respiratory distress syndrome. Am J Respir Crit Care Med 1994; 149(2):295–305.

This study showed no advantage to low-flow extracorporeal CO_2 removal (including the learning curve for that technique) when compared with the results of carefully controlled conventional management, with a 60% mortality in both groups.

Murray JF, Matthay MA, Luce JM, Flick MR. Pulmonary perspectives. An expanded definition of the adult respiratory distress syndrome. Am Rev Respir Dis 1988; 138:720–3.

This report includes the "Murray score" of ARDS.

Niehoff J, Delguercio C, LaMorte W, et al. Efficacy of pulse oximetry and capnometry in postoperative ventilatory weaning. Crit Care Med 1988;16:701–5.
A typical study showing the advantages of continuous end-tidal CO_2 monitoring in critically ill patients.

Parker JC, Hernandez LA, Peevy KJ. Mechanisms of ventilator induced lung injury. Crit Care Med 1993;21:131–43.

Parker JC, Townsley MI, Rippe J. Increased microvascular permeability in dogs due to high peak airway pressures. J Appl Physiol 1984;57:1809–16.
These two papers describe capillary and alveolar high-pressure (overdistention) lung injury.

Pelosi P, D'Andrea L, Vitale G, Pesenti A, Gattinoni L. Vertical gradient of regional lung inflation in adult respiratory distress syndrome. Am J Respir Crit Care Med 1994;149:8–13.
Definition of the regional distribution of water and dependent lung consolidation in ARDS.

Potkin RT, Swenson ER. Resuscitation from severe acute hypercapnia. Determinants of tolerance and survival. Chest 1992;102:1742–5.
A case report of a patient who had a P_{CO_2} of 375 mm Hg and pH of 6.6. The patient was comatose but had an uneventful recovery after undergoing appropriate ventilator treatment. This is one of many articles that demonstrates the benign nature of respiratory acidosis.

Pratt PC, Vollmer RT, Shelburne JD, Crapo JD. Pulmonary morphology in a multi-hospital collaborative extracorporeal membrane oxygenation project. Am J Pathol 1979;95:191–214.
Histologic characteristics of ARDS gleaned from the first NIH-extracorporeal membrane oxygenation study.

Rodriguez JL, Steinberg SM, Luchetti FA, et al. Early tracheostomy for primary airway management in the surgical critical care setting. Surgery 1990;108:655–9.
Early tracheostomy was associated with a lowered incidence of pneumonia in trauma and critical care patients.

Severinghaus JW, Bradley AF. Electrodes for blood P_{O_2} and P_{CO_2} determination. J Appl Physiol 1958;13:515–20.
The original description of the Severinghaus P_{CO_2} electrode

Simmons RS, Berdine GG, Seidenfeld JJ, et al. Fluid balance in the adult respiratory distress syndrome. Am Rev Respir Dis 1987;135:924–9.
This study of 113 patients with ARDS show that survival was much improved in patients who had a significant negative fluid balance during their ICU stay. Although this was not a prospective randomized study, it clearly defines a rationale for achieving dry weight in such patients.

Slutsky AS. Mechanical ventilation. The ACCP consensus conference. Chest 1993;104:1833–59.
A large panel chaired by Arthur Slutsky defined many aspects of mechanical ventilation, including general recommendations for the safe use of mechanical ventilators.

Starling EH. The influence of mechanical factors on lymph production. J Physiol 1894;16:224.
The original description of Starling's equation for determining transcapillary flux.

Vasilyev S, Schaap RN, Mortensen JD. Hospital survival rates of patients with acute respiratory failure in the modern respiratory intensive care unit: an international, multi-center, prospective survey. Chest 1995;107:1083–88.

A 12-center study of the epidemiology and natural history of acute respiratory failure in adults. In 1991 the mortality in all categories was decreased by about 20% compared with the 1986 figure.

Zapol WM, Frikker MJ, Pontoppidian H, Wilson RS, Lynch KE. The adult respiratory distress syndrome at the Massachusetts General Hospital: etiology, progression and survival rates, 1978–88. In: Zapol WM, Lamare F, eds. Adult respiratory distress syndrome. New York: Dekker, 1991.

This epidemiologically oriented paper is included in a very good multi-authored review of ARDS. The Massachusetts General Hospital series and scoring system is described.

4

Metabolism and Nutrition

Metabolic Requirements

The typical expenditures of energy and protein in normal subjects and critically ill patients are shown in Figure 4-1. Protein and energy requirements are continuous. These are met by endogenous sources during fasting or can be met through exogenous treatment (nutrition). Energy expenditure is referred to as the *basal metabolic rate* or the *basal energy expenditure* and represents a near-sleep steady state. More commonly we refer to the *resting energy expenditure* (REE) measured after a brief period of supine rest. The REE is properly expressed in joules, the standard unit of energy, but is more commonly and more practically expressed in calories. The REE decreases with advancing age and varies with sex and body size. It is a function of cellular metabolism, and hence of the body cell mass (Figure 4-2). The REE is usually estimated from a chart combining age, sex, and body size data. Such charts are based on or are similar to those originally published by Harris and Benedict.

Estimating and Measuring Energy Requirements

The actual metabolic rate of any given patient can be estimated by taking the predicted basal rate and adjusting it according to that expected in the setting of the patient's particular clinical condition. For example, the metabolic rate is typically decreased by 10% in a starving person and increased by 10% with minor activity. Trauma, stress, sepsis, and surgical operations are all known to cause the metabolic rate to increase. Several authors have proposed tables or formulas for estimating the metabolic rate depending on the degree of physiologic stress (Figures 4-3 and 4-4). This amount of energy is most

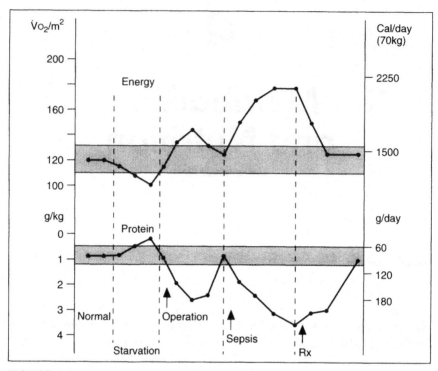

FIGURE 4-1. Energy and protein expenditure in the setting of common clinical conditions. The normal daily expenditure is shown in the shaded area. (From: Bartlett RH. In Dantzker D (ed). Cardiopulmonary Critical Care. New York: Grune & Stratton, 1986.)

conveniently expressed in calories per day (Table 4-1). The metabolic rate is normalized to the body surface area; however, the actively metabolizing tissue is actually the lean body cell mass. Consequently, reporting the rate in "per square meter" units underestimates metabolism in a fat person and overestimates it in a very lean person.

Although most of the studies on nutrition in the setting of critical illness have been based on the estimated energy expenditure, actual measurement is much more accurate and is becoming an important aspect of critical care management. The most commonly used method of measurement is indirect calorimetry. In this method the amount of oxygen absorbed across the lungs into the pulmonary blood is measured over a given period. Assuming the patient is at a metabolic steady state during this time, the amount of oxygen absorbed across the lungs is equal to the amount of oxygen consumed in the metabolic processes. (This is the basic assumption of the Fick equation and is the reason why oxygen consumption is a valid measurement of metabolism, even in patients with abnormal lung function.) The energy released through the oxidation of various food substrates is known from direct

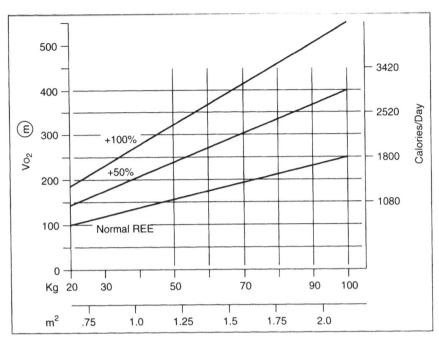

FIGURE 4-2. Resting energy expenditure (REE) related to size.

measurements, so that the metabolic rate measured in cubic centimeters of oxygen per minute can be converted to calories per hour or per day if the oxygenated substrates are known. For practical purposes, a conversion factor of 5 kcal of energy per liter of oxygen consumed is a reasonable approximation. It overestimates the metabolic rate slightly but the rate yielded is a much more accurate approximation of the actual metabolic rate than is a number derived from an arbitrary chart or table.

Energy Sources

The major sources of energy are carbohydrates (including ketones and alcohols) and fats. Protein can be oxidized and is often an important source of energy in critically ill patients (Table 4-2). In nutritional planning we strive to supply energy from nonprotein sources, allowing the use of endogenous and exogenous proteins for anabolism rather than for catabolism. In both normal subjects and surgical patients, protein breakdown is decreased by the administration of exogenous fuel, be it glucose, fat, or xylitol. This is referred to as the *protein-sparing effect*. Small amounts of glucose (400 cal/day) provide some protein sparing, but full caloric support is required for maximal effect.

Carbohydrate is the major source of energy under normal, nonstarving conditions. The brain, the red blood cells, and possibly other tissues are all

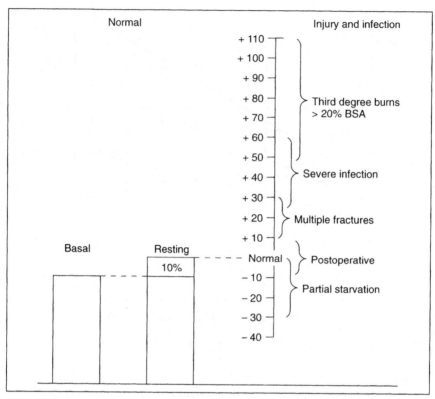

FIGURE 4-3. Changes in resting energy expenditure associated with common clinical conditions, as diagrammed by Kinney. (BSA = body surface area.) (From: Kinney JM. Energy requirements of the surgical patients. In: The American College of Surgeons manual, surgical nutrition. Philadelphia: Saunders, 1975.)

obligate glucose users. They require glucose as the primary energy source under normal conditions. Other organs also use glucose preferentially as a source of energy. The brain and red blood cells can develop the capacity to use ketones as an energy source, a process called *starvation adaptation*. When fully oxidized, carbohydrate produces 4.0 cal of energy per gram of substrate, 5.0 cal of energy per liter of oxygen consumed, and one molecule of CO_2 for each molecule of oxygen consumed. The latter ratio is the respiratory quotient (RQ), which is 1.0 for carbohydrate (Table 4-3).

Fat is the most efficient source of energy: It produces 9 cal of energy per gram of substrate metabolized and 4.7 cal per liter of oxygen consumed in this oxidation, and has an RQ of 0.7. Fat is stored as triglyceride, and for each three molecules of fatty acid oxidized to produce energy, one molecule of glycerol is also oxidized. Endogenous fat is the major source of energy during starvation. The glycogen stores are basically depleted after a day of fasting, and fat becomes the major source of energy, always with protein breakdown.

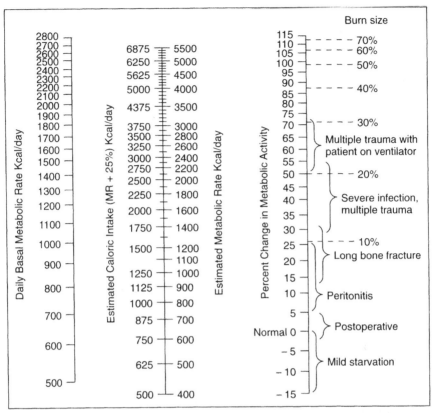

FIGURE 4-4. Changes in resting energy expenditure associated with common clinical conditions, as diagrammed by Wilmore. Using a straight line, connect the normal basal metabolic rate on the left (25 kcal/kg /day) to the clinical condition on the right. Read the estimated caloric requirement from the column in the middle. (MR = metabolic rate.) (From: Wilmore DW. The metabolic management of the critically ill. New York: Plenum, 1977.)

TABLE 4-1. Nutrition and Metabolism

Energy Variable	Normal Value
$\dot{V}O_2$	100–130 cc ⓜ STPD
$\dot{V}CO_2$	80–130 cc ⓜ STPD
RQ	$\dot{V}CO_2/\dot{V}O_2$
REE	25 cal/kg/day; 960 cal/ⓜ/day
BEE	20 cal/kg/day; 800 cal/ⓜ/day
Caloric balance	Calories in − REE (measured)
$\dot{V}O_2$/calorie conversion: $\dot{V}O_2$ L/min × 60 min × 24 h × 5 cal/L = cal/day (same as $\dot{V}O_2$ × 7200)	

BEE = basal energy expenditure; ⓜ = min/m²; REE = resting energy expenditure; RQ = respiratory quotient; STPD = standard pressure, temperature, dry; $\dot{V}CO_2$ = CO_2 production; $\dot{V}O_2$ = oxygen consumption.

TABLE 4-2. Protein Metabolism*

1 g of nitrogen = 6.25 g of protein
Nitrogen loss: 5–10 g/day, 85% as urea
Protein catabolic rate
Normal: 0.5–1 g/kg/day
Hypercatabolic = 1.5–2 g/kg/day

*Protein metabolism is measured and described in terms of the elemental nitrogen gain or loss.

TABLE 4-3. Characteristics of Oxidation of Three Classes of Substrates

Substrate	Calories per Gram	Respiratory Quotient	Calories per Liter of Oxygen
Carbohydrate	4	1.0	5
Fat	9	0.7	4.75
Protein	4	0.8	4.8

Mediators

The identity and actions of mediators of the hypermetabolic state are incompletely known. Elevated catecholamine levels have been identified in burn patients. Corticosteroids, glucagon, growth hormone, and thyroid hormone have all been implicated as mediators of the hypermetabolic state in various critical conditions. Interleukin-2 causes both hypermetabolism and protein catabolism. Certain amino acids may play a modulating role. Alanine, for example, has easy access to the gluconeogenetic pathway, and it has been suggested that protein catabolism is dependent on the amount of alanine produced. Fischer and others have shown that infusing patients with branched-chain amino acids diminishes protein catabolism and have proposed the use of solutions rich in branched-chain amino acids for the treatment of patients in catabolic states. Whatever the mediator of the hypermetabolic state is, it appears best to treat the underlying cause while feeding metabolic fuel to the fire rather than attempting to reverse the hypermetabolism per se.

Protein Metabolism

Estimating and Measuring Protein Requirements

In normal protein metabolism there is a continuous excretion of nitrogen (mostly as urea) equivalent to approximately 50 g of protein each day, matched by a protein intake of 50 g/day.

The protein synthesis and breakdown rate is approximately 300 g/day, with most endogenous amino acids being recycled into new protein. Under starvation conditions, protein catabolism continues (although at a slower rate) without a corresponding protein intake, leaving the patient in a negative protein balance. This protein flux is most conveniently measured as nitrogen flux; consequently this condition is commonly referred to as a *negative nitrogen balance*. During critical illness the rate of protein catabolism generally increases while intake stops, resulting in a negative nitrogen balance. It is convenient to think of this protein breakdown as "necessary" for producing more glucose through the gluconeogenetic pathway when other carbohydrate stores have been exhausted.

Protein Sources

The fact that the nitrogen balance is negative does not mean that protein synthesis stops or slows down. On the contrary, new tissues, inflammatory cells, collagen, coagulation factors, antibodies, and scores of other proteins are synthesized at an accelerated rate during critical illness. Amino acids derived from muscle tissue or other somatic and visceral proteins become the building blocks for protein in healing tissue and host defenses. The site of a traumatic or surgical wound or area of acute inflammation becomes a protein "parasite" on other body tissues. Eventually this "parasite" may overwhelm the host, because proteins that would otherwise go to strengthening the diaphragm or the myocardium or participate in host defense processes are thrown to the metabolic flames. A large part of the goal of nutritional management therefore is to provide energy sources so that endogenous proteins are not required for energy (that is, protein sparing) and to supply exogenous proteins such that all the needs of protein synthesis can be met without the breaking down of endogenous sources. Although oversimplified, a convenient number to remember for the basal protein requirement is 1 g/kg/day or 40 g/m^2/day.

Mediators

The mediators of protein catabolism appear to differ from the mediators of the metabolic rate. Although energy requirement and protein breakdown often follow similar patterns, there are patients who have major protein catabolism at a normal metabolic rate and patients who are hypermetabolic while conserving protein. Tumor necrosis factor is a specific mediator released from monocytes that stimulates endogenous protein breakdown. This is corroborated by clinical observations in which the degree of protein catabolism generally correlates with the degree of inflammation and (presumed) neutrophil and monocyte activation.

TABLE 4-4. Typical Adult Daily Requirements for Vitamins and Trace Metals

Substance	Requirement
Vitamin A	3,300 IU
Vitamin C	100 mg
Vitamin D	200 IU
Vitamin E	10 IU
Thiamine B_1	3 mg
Riboflavin B_2	3 mg
Pyridoxine B_6	4 mg
Pyridoxine B_{12}	5 μcg
Niacin	40 mg
Pantothenic Acid	15 mg
Biotin	60 μcg
Folic acid	410 μcg
Calcium	15 mEq
Magnesium	20 mEq
Phosphorus	50 mmol/L
Zinc	5 mg
Copper	1 mg
Manganese	0.5 mg
Chromium	0.01 mg
Selenium	0.06 mg
Linoleic Acid	1 g

Vitamins and Minerals

Vitamin stores are plentiful and deficiency states develop slowly, so vitamin loss is not a concern during the early days of critical illness. A hypermetabolic patient catabolizes vitamins more rapidly than a normal person does and can reach a deficiency state sooner. A patient who is severely malnourished before admittance to the intensive care unit (ICU) may already have a vitamin deficiency. There is some evidence that high doses of vitamins A and C may be beneficial to patients with injuries. Because vitamins are inexpensive and safe, we approach vitamin therapy in the ICU in the same way as we do in the clinic—prescribe more than enough for the patient who is not eating. Commercial preparations for enteral or parenteral use provide gross excesses of vitamins but do not lead to overdose.

Trace metals must be managed more carefully than vitamins because deficiency can occur sooner and overdose can be deleterious. Calcium, phosphorus, magnesium, and sulfur are more than trace elements. They are lost continuously in the urine, stool, gastric juices, and other drainage fluids. Although there are large body stores (particularly of calcium and phosphorus), deficiency can develop rapidly. Enteral and parenteral feeding must therefore include these elements. Serum levels of calcium, phosphorus, and magnesium should be measured at regular intervals. Zinc, copper, chromium, selenium, and manganese must be supplied to patients who are supported with enteral or parenteral feeding for more than 2 weeks. Recommended daily allowances for vitamins and trace minerals are listed in Table 4-4.

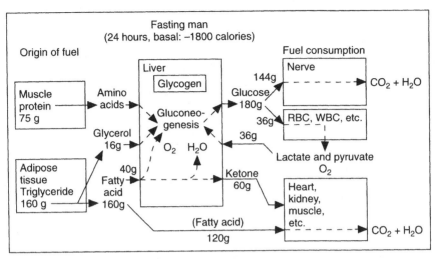

FIGURE 4-5. Metabolic events after one day of starvation in a normal human being. (From: Cahill G. Starvation in man. N Engl J Med 1970; 282:668–75.)

Endogenous Sources of Energy and Protein

In a normal 80-kg man, approximately 1000 cal are available in the form of glycogen and other stored carbohydrates. About 140,000 cal are stored as fat. The body contains approximately 6 kg of protein, which could be either consumed as an energy source or maintained to do work. Nutritional assessment is the process of measuring the amount of these energy and protein reserves.

Almost all critically ill patients are starving (have no caloric or protein intake) unless we supply feeding for them. Because starvation is such an integral part of the physiologic status of a critical care patient, it is a very instructive exercise to calculate the sources, fate, and balance of fat, carbohydrate, and protein in a normal but starving person. Fortunately George Cahill has done this for us and published the results in a classic article several years ago. The metabolic consequences of starving for 24 hours as described by Cahill are shown in Figure 4-5. After 24 hours of starvation, the liver and muscle glycogen store has been depleted and the glucose utilized in metabolism is generated from fat, protein, and lactate in the process of gluconeogenesis. The amount of glucose generated in this process is 180 g. At 4 cal per gram this process supplies 720 cal worth of energy, most of which is used up in nervous system metabolism. The remaining 60% of the energy substrate is supplied by ketone bodies and fatty acids resulting from fat breakdown. This source of energy is more than twice as efficient as gluconeogenesis (expressed as calories per gram), as anyone who has tried to lose body fat through starvation can attest to. Notice that the protein catabolic rate is 1 g/kg/day, and remember that this is the rate for a normal person, not a hypermetabolic, critically ill patient.

110 Critical Care Physiology

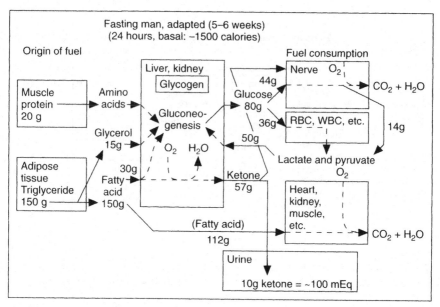

FIGURE 4-6. Metabolic events after five weeks of starvation in a normal human being. (From: Cahill G. Starvation in man. N Engl J Med 1970;282:668–75.)

If starvation goes untreated, there is a gradual shift in the types of substrates supplying the energy for metabolism. This shift occurs because enzymes in nervous tissue are induced to act on ketone in addition to glucose as a major energy source. This adaptation decreases the need for gluconeogenesis, so that the protein breakdown that was necessary to supply glucose can be considerably curtailed. These adjustments represent a marvelous bit of teleologic biology, because the chronically starving person would otherwise rapidly become too weak to move or breathe if protein catabolism continued at its usual rate. Starvation adaptation facilitates protein, and therefore muscle mass, conservation. The metabolic events in this adaptation process were also calculated for us by Cahill and are shown in Figure 4-6. Once a person is adapted to fasting, the resting energy expenditure has decreased from 1800 to 1500 cal per day, presumably because the chronically starving man is much less active. In starvation adaptation, 40% of the caloric energy still goes to the nervous system and blood cells, but only half of that energy is supplied by gluconeogenesis and the balance is furnished by ketones derived from fat. Fat catabolism continues at almost the same rate as it did after 24 hours of fasting, but muscle catabolism decreases from 75 to 20 g per day. Although protein breakdown is considerably decreased in starvation adaptation, it never goes to zero. This "protein floor" (usually expressed as 2 g of nitrogen or 12 g of protein per day) represents the least amount of protein intake that is compatible with life over a period of weeks or months. Remember that the critically ill patient may indeed be in a state of starvation adaptation, but often other factors such as inflammation are operating that override this adaptive mechanism and produce major increases rather than decreases in the protein catabolic rate.

Energy Reserves

The simplest way of measuring nutritional status is to determine the body weight in relation to height. Major changes in weight that are not caused by fluid shifts are related to changes in the amount of body fat. Energy reserves are generally estimated in terms of the amount of body fat, as the amount of carbohydrate held in reserve is negligible. The first approach to measuring the energy reserve is to estimate the caloric balance. The daily REE is estimated as already discussed, and the daily energy intake is estimated from the caloric value of the nutrients taken in daily. The latter estimate is easy to do for critically ill patients because such patients are usually receiving nothing by mouth and all calories are supplied through parenteral or tube feeding routes. A 10,000-cal deficit in a critically ill patient is a severe, acute energy deficit, although this represents only 5 or 6 days of semistarvation. The problem associated with a 10,000-cal deficit is not the loss of a few kilograms of fat, but rather the associated protein catabolism that is commonly associated with this degree of an energy deficit. Fat reserves can be estimated by measuring the thickness of the triceps skin fold or by examining changes in body weight, corrected for fluid balance. Measurement of arm circumference includes both fat and muscle mass. Any of these measurements of body fat represent at best a gross approximation.

Protein Reserve

Because protein is the functional and structural chemical of the body, most nutritional assessment techniques are estimations of protein reserves. The creatinine/height index is basically a measurement of the amount of creatinine excreted (as a measure of muscle breakdown), normalized for body size. Because muscle is a major source of endogenous protein, muscle wasting is characteristic of the malnourished state. This can be detected by muscle strength and endurance testing. There are a few standardized methods of muscle testing that are used for nutritional assessment. One such test is the measurement of the maximal breathing capacity (also known as the *maximal voluntary ventilation*). In this test the maximal amount of air that can be moved by means of rapid breathing during 12 seconds is measured. The values are expressed as the percentage of the predicted amount for a given age, sex, and size (normal is 80% to 120%). In the absence of significant obstructive or restrictive disease, a low value usually indicates a lack of muscle strength and endurance. Inspiratory force is another strength test that is easily and commonly done in the ICU. The normal range is 80 to 100 cm H_2O.

The actual nitrogen balance can be determined by measuring the amount of nitrogen excreted. This is most conveniently done by measuring the amount of urea excreted in the urine, assuming that urea constitutes 85% of the total nitrogen excretion. However, it is better to actually measure the total nitrogen content in urine and other fluid losses, because the proportion of urea may vary considerably. Once the nitrogen excretion level is known, the amount of protein catabolized can be estimated and compared with the amount of protein ingested by the patient. Indirect assessments of protein reserves are based on a single measurement of body substances that are dependent on rapid protein synthesis for the maintenance of normal levels. Levels of conventional serum proteins such as albumin and globulin are not affected by malnutrition until it is very severe. Levels of proteins such as prealbumin and transferrin, which turn over more rapidly, are better indicators of protein status. Lymphocytes are rapidly destroyed, and protein is required for the formation of new cells. Consequently the absolute lymphocyte count is a useful measure of the status of protein reserves. The lymphocyte count, in our experience, is the best single "static" measurement for characterizing nutritional status.

Protein is also required for synthesizing the cells and mediators involved in skin test reactivity. Although skin test reactivity is a manifestation of lymphocyte-mediated immunity, its usefulness in patient evaluation is probably due to its ability to assess the inflammatory response rather than lymphocyte activity per se. The McGill surgical research group showed, for example, that neutrophil chemotaxis (or the lack of it) correlates with the degree of cutaneous sensitivity to recall antigens. Some chronically and acutely malnourished patients convert from reactive to anergic, and reactivity can be restored by nutritional repletion.

These methods of nutritional assessment are used to determine the nutritional status of patients at the time of injury, operation, or critical illness (Table 4-5). The most important markers are listed in Table 4-6.

In those patients who are suffering from both energy and protein depletion at the time of major physiologic stress, the morbidity and mortality are higher than they are in those whose nutritional status is normal. Preoperative nutritional treatment is associated with a decrease in postoperative morbidity and mortality in high-risk, malnourished patients. Measurements of fat reserves are not helpful during the acute management of critically ill patients. Measurements of protein reserves are somewhat helpful but cannot reflect hour-to-hour or day-to-day metabolic changes. In an excellent study the McGill group measured body cell mass (the gold standard way of assessing nutritional status) and found that the depleted state could not be reliably detected on the basis of the weight/height index, the triceps skin fold, the midarm circumference, the albumin level, the total protein level, hand

TABLE 4-5. Measurement of Nutritional Reserves

			Depletion	
Reserve	Excess	Normal	Mild	Severe
Energy reserves				
Cumulative caloric balance (cal)	+	0	−5,000	−10,000
Triceps skin fold (%)	−	Per table	−5	−40
Arm circumference (%)	−	Per table	−5	−30
Weight change (%)	−	Variable	−5	−20
Protein reserves				
Creatinine/height index (%)		Per table	−5	−30
Lymphocyte count (/mm^3)	>2,000	1800	1600	500
Cumulative nitrogen balance (g)	+	0	−30	−300
Albumin (g/dL)	>3	3	2.5	1.5
Prealbumin (mg/dL)	>20	20	10.0	5.0
Total protein (g/dL)	>8	6	5.5	4.0
Muscle strength				
Inspiratory force (cm H$_2$O)	>100	200	50	20
Maximal volume ventilation (% predicted)	>120	100	60	30
Skin test reactivity		Reactive	Anergic	

TABLE 4-6. Markers of Acute Nutritional Status

Marker	Values Showing Depletion	Normal Value
Lymphocytes (/mm^3)	<1500	3000
Cumulative caloric balance (cal)	−10,000	0
Cumulative protein balance (g)	−500	0
Albumin (g/dL)	<3	>3
Prealbumin (mg/dL)	<10	>20

strength, or the creatinine/height ratio. Actual measurements of metabolic rate and nitrogen balance are the best way of monitoring nutritional status in critically ill patients.

Energy and Protein Balance

Energy expenditure is most conveniently measured using the techniques of respirometry and indirect calorimetry discussed in detail in Chapters 1 and 3. Direct volumetric spirometry is the best method for measuring oxygen consumption. This technique also lends itself well to the simultaneous measurement of CO_2 production. The RQ can be calculated from the oxygen consumption and CO_2 production values.

The relative amounts of carbohydrate and fat that are oxidized can be calculated from the RQ. The RQ for protein is 0.8. By measuring the urinary nitrogen level, the amount of protein catabolized can be calculated and the measured RQ can be "corrected" for the amount of oxygen and CO_2 involved in protein catabolism. For example, if the urinary nitrogen excretion rate is 0.5 g/hr, then protein has been metabolized at a rate of 3 g/hr, accounting for 3200 mL of oxygen consumed per hour and 2560 mL of CO_2 produced per hour. This "nonprotein" RQ is used to define the amount of fat or carbohydrate used as energy sources. Ketones have a very low RQ (0.6), so that ketone metabolism will cause the overall RQ to be lower. On the other hand, the conversion of glucose to fat generates CO_2, so that the RQ of this reaction is more than 1.0. Measurement of the RQ is helpful as an internal check of the accuracy of the calorimetric measurements and as a guideline to patient management. For example, if a patient has been receiving only 500 cal/day and has a metabolic rate of 2500 cal/day, one would expect that fat utilization would be maximum and the RQ should be between 0.7 and 0.8. If such a patient is treated with parenteral nutrition utilizing glucose as the major source of energy, the RQ should be 1.0 when the caloric replacement matches caloric losses. If the RQ exceeds 1.0, then some of the infused carbohydrate is being converted to fat, producing an excess amount of CO_2 that increases the need for breathing. Hypercaloric feeding with glucose can lead to respiratory failure requiring mechanical ventilation simply by increasing the load of CO_2. Determining the energy balance is helpful because it serves to identify the high-risk patient. In our studies, the mortality was much higher in acutely ill patients with caloric deficits greater than 10,000 cal than it was in those patients with a positive caloric balance.

A typical balance diagram is shown in Figure 4-7. In this diagram the intake during a 24-hour period is plotted from the baseline up and expenditures are plotted from that point back down toward the baseline. In the example shown in this figure, the intake was 2000 cal worth of food stuffs and the expenditure was exactly 2000 cal, resulting in a zero balance for that day. On the next day the intake was 2000 cal but the expenditure was only 1600 cal, resulting in a 400-cal positive balance. On the third day the intake was 1000 cal and the expenditure was 2000 cal, making the cumulative balance a deficit of 600 cal. The fourth day is total starvation. With no caloric intake and 2000 cal expended, the cumulative balance is now a deficit of 2600 cal. Balance diagrams like this can and should be constructed for critically ill patients for all variables that are crucial to effective patient management, including the energy substrate, protein, water, sodium, potassium, and other electrolytes in some cases. The metabolic steps involved in protein metabolism are diagrammed in a different way in Figure 4-8. When renal function is normal, almost all the products of protein catabolism appear as nitrogen compounds in the urine, so that measuring the total urinary nitrogen level provides a direct measure of the net protein balance. Notice that the actual rate of protein turnover in muscle, liver, and kidney is much higher than the net rate of protein loss.

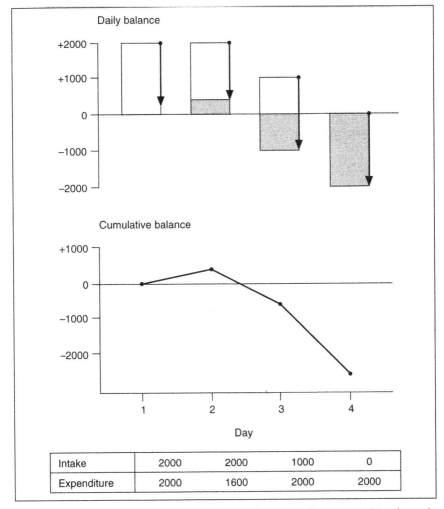

FIGURE 4-7. Energy balance for a 70-kg adult ranging from normal intake and metabolism (day 1) to starvation (day 4).

In renal failure, by-products of protein catabolism accumulate in the body rather than appearing in the urine. Although urea is not the only metabolite of protein breakdown, its level is the one most easily measured. To calculate the net protein breakdown in renal failure it is necessary to measure the urea nitrogen concentration in blood at the beginning and end of a timed period. Then, along with some assumptions regarding the extracellular fluid volume and the distribution of urea and other protein breakdown products in extracellular fluid, it is possible to calculate a "protein catabolic rate" that

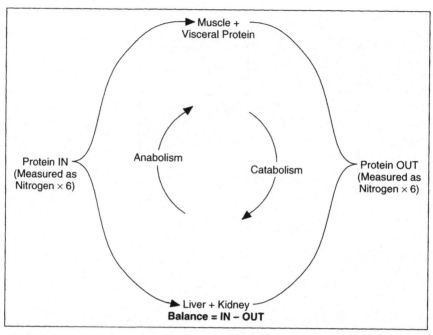

FIGURE 4-8. Events leading to protein breakdown and calculation of the net loss.

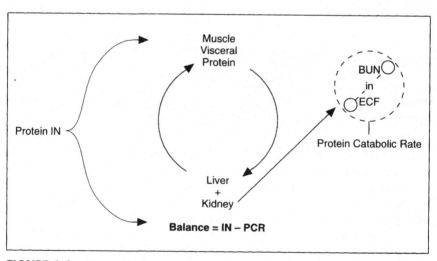

FIGURE 4-9. Events leading to protein breakdown in renal failure and calculation of the net loss. (BUN = blood urea nitrogen; ECF = extracellular fluid; PCR = protein catabolic rate.)

approximates the net protein loss despite the fact that there is no urine (Figure 4-9). The method for making this calculation was developed by Sargent.

Nutrition Supplies

Energy and Protein

The goal of nutritional therapy in critically ill patients is to maintain a positive nitrogen balance and to prevent endogenous protein breakdown. Exogenous protein can be given by means of the gastrointestinal (GI) tract or parenterally. Parenteral administration usually makes use of amino acid solutions, although peptide solutions may be adequate for most conditions. The amino acid compositions of commercially available enteral and parenteral feeding solutions are arbitrarily designed. The original amino acid solution was concocted to resemble hens' egg albumin, for example. The "best" combination of amino acids has not been determined and probably differs for different disease states.

The interrelationship between the amount of protein and the amount of energy supplied to the patient is a matter of some discussion. In the steady state a 70-kg adult typically consumes 1800 cal and 60 g of protein each day, for a ratio of 30 cal/g of protein or 187 cal/g of nitrogen. This would be the appropriate amount of nutrients for a patient who is not nutritionally depleted and is not hypermetabolic—for example, a patient with Guillain-Barré syndrome who is on ventilator support. If the patient is nutritionally depleted but not hypermetabolic (for example, a patient with esophageal cancer being prepared for operation), the maximal amount of protein that can be "loaded into" the active body cell mass should be given. The actual amount depends on the simultaneous caloric support, because a greater positive nitrogen balance can be achieved with a given nitrogen supply when a positive caloric balance is achieved at the same time (Figure 4-10). In such a patient it would be appropriate to give 150 g of protein and 2500 cal daily (a ratio of 13 cal/g of protein or 85 cal/g of nitrogen), realizing that, if the bulk of the calories are given in the form of carbohydrate, some of this carbohydrate will be converted to fat, thus producing CO_2 and raising the minute ventilation requirement. A patient who is actively catabolizing protein because of depleted carbohydrate energy stores combined with a hypermetabolic state (for example, a major burn patient) requires an energy supply to match his or her hypermetabolic losses (for example, 3500 cal in a burn patient who is metabolizing 3000 cal/day). An exogenous supply of energy may slow down or turn off protein catabolism, but it also may not; therefore it is the current practice to provide gross excesses of protein to these patients. Such a patient would typically receive 3500 mL of a 4% protein formula, hence 140 g of protein with 3500 cal, or a ratio of 25 cal/g of protein (160 cal/g of nitrogen).

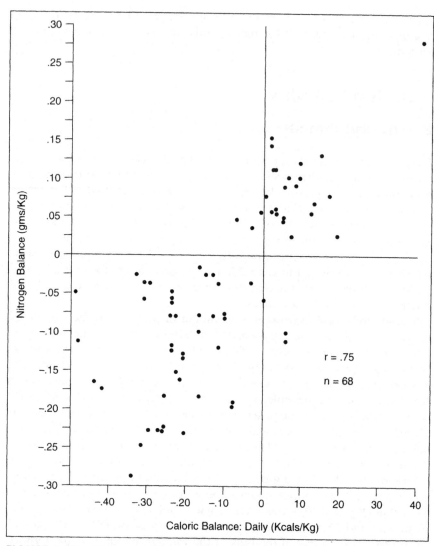

FIGURE 4-10. Nitrogen balance related to energy balance in critically ill patients treated with standard parenteral nutrition solutions with 40 g of amino acid and 1000 cal of glucose per liter. (Author's data.)

Methods of Supplying Nutrition

Feeding by mouth is the most efficient way of providing energy and protein and is feasible in many critically ill patients. Giving patients milk shakes, eggnog, solid candy, or popsicles is better than giving them water or fruit juices, as is the common practice in critical care units. The possibility of oral feeding is one of several reasons why tracheostomy is preferable to endotracheal intubation for the long-term management of patients with acute respiratory failure.

Enteral Feeding

If the patient cannot or will not take food by mouth, liquid food should be administered directly into the stomach or intestine through a feeding tube.

Enteral feeding can be accomplished by a tube passed directly into the duodenum or jejunum at operation or by a tube passed into the stomach through the nose or mouth. Soft, small-bore feeding catheters with weighted tips are commercially available, but small-bore nasogastric tubes can serve just as well. It is generally possible to accomplish tube feeding with gastric infusion. Patients with gastric ileus, such as those who have just undergone abdominal operations, can be fed into the jejunum during the period of gastric atony.

Formulas for tube feeding range from milk to commercial preparations. Although milk with supplements or blenderized hospital diet food is probably the most economical tube-feeding formula, standardized commercial preparations are the most widely used because they are easy to prepare and sterile and the composition is precisely known. These commercial preparations range from 1.0 to 2 cal/mL and protein makes up 3% to 7% of their composition. Most of the calories are supplied as glucose or sucrose, so that the solutions have a high osmolarity. Cramps or diarrhea can result when these high-osmolarity solutions are placed into the stomach or intestine. Diarrhea is the major complication associated with most tube-feeding formulations, and it can usually be controlled by adding pectin to the feedings. A large amount of pectin may be required. Diarrhea can also be minimized by using starch or fat as an energy source in tube feedings. This can be supplied as part of the commercial preparation or added in the form of medium-chain triglycerides or other oils. The best results are usually achieved by supplying approximately half of the calories as carbohydrate and half as fat. Although some formulations are advertised as "low residue," almost all the liquid feeding formulas are completely absorbed in the small intestine. Typical formulas are listed in Table 4-7. Whatever formulation is used, there are some tricks to using enteral feeding that are often neglected, with the result that regurgitation or diarrhea occurs and the feedings are terminated. Feedings should be given by continuous infusion into the stomach extending over

24 hours rather than as large boluses. It is rarely necessary to give more than 100 mL/hr. When possible, the patient should be in a sitting position (or in a side-to-side, head-up position) to prevent regurgitation along the tube. Gastric residuals should be checked if the patient feels uncomfortable or appears distended, but it is not necessary to check the residual more than once a day. With continuous tube feeding a residual of 200 to 300 mL is normal.

It is usually recommended that the patient be started on 50 mL/hr of a diluted (half-strength) feeding formula, followed by an increase in the volume and then the concentration of the formula until 100 to 150 mL/hr of full-strength formula is reached. In my experience, it is better to start with a small amount of full-strength formula rather than a large amount of diluted formula. The amount (rather than the concentration) should be increased gradually until the desired volume is reached. Tube feedings can be supplemented by oral intake. The intake of popsicles, hard candy, peanut butter, eggnog, and the like should be encouraged. The volume of feedings can be decreased proportionate to the number of calories taken in by mouth. As already noted, diarrhea can almost always be controlled by the administration of pectin. Hypernatremia can result if the tube feeding is rich in sodium. This should be managed by the administration of low-salt solutions or free water. A serious problem with tube feeding is the complete cessation of feedings by the nursing staff when diarrhea or a high gastric residual occurs. If the tube feeding needs to be curtailed for any reason, it should be reinstituted the next hour at a smaller volume and the volume gradually increased until the prescribed caloric load is reached again.

Feeding formulas support bacterial growth, and sometimes the diarrhea and cramps represent "food poisoning." The food should be prepared fresh daily and refrigerated until used. A new aliquot should be started every 8 to 12 hours.

Tube Feeding to Prevent Intestinal Atrophy and Cholestasis

Twenty-five years ago, hypermetabolic, critically ill patients who could not be fed died. With the development of total parenteral nutrition by Dudrick and his colleagues, we began to see patients who lived for weeks while supported by parenteral feeding alone. Many of these patients recovered from their primary disease, were eventually able to eat normally again, and are alive today because of parenteral nutrition. Along with this marvelous progress came the recognition of intestinal mucosal atrophy and cholestasis, both of which commonly occurred in patients on total parenteral support for more than a few days. There is good evidence that the loss of mucosal thickness in these patients invites the absorption of bacterial toxins or intact bacteria. This endogenous source of chronic inflammation compounded by compromised liver function has been postulated as the underlying mechanism responsible for the multiple-organ failure often seen in patients who go without enteric feeding for a long period. Throughout the development of parenteral feeding it has been documented many times that enteral feeding with equivalent substrates is always better than parenteral feeding. ("Better

TABLE 4-7. Typical Feeding Formulas

TPN Solution	Carbohydrate (%)	Fat (%)	Protein (%)	mOsm/L	cal/L	Sodium (mEq/L)	Potassium (mEq/L)	Other
Parenteral								
10% Glucose	10	0	4.25	880	440	47	23	36 mEq acetate
25% Glucose	25	0	4.25	1825	1020	35	40	25 mEq acetate
10% Lipid	—	10	—	276	1000	0	0	—
Enteral*								
Criticare HN	22	0.3	3.8	650	1060	27	34	Tube only
Osmolyte HN	14.1	3.7	4.4	310	1060	40	40	Tube only
Isocal	12.6	4.2	3.2	300	1060	22	32	Tube only
Ensure	14.5	3.7	3.7	470	1060	37	40	Orally or tube
Jevity	15.2	3.7	4.4	310	1060	41	40	Tube only
Replete	11.3	3.3	6.2	350	1000	22	40	Orally or tube

TPN = total parenteral nutrition.
*Commercial names are used.

than" here means better liver function, less organ failure, better endurance, and better host defenses as observed in laboratory animals.) This usually translates into a shorter ICU stay, fewer complications, and perhaps better survival in critically ill patients fed enterally rather than parenterally. Some, if not all, of the advantages of enteral feeding can be attributed to the prevention of intestinal mucosal atrophy and cholestasis. Recent evidence indicates that the mucosal atrophy can be prevented by the administration of small amounts of the amino acid glutamine into the lumen of the intestine. It is interesting to note that all enteral feeding formulas contain glutamine but standard amino acid formulas used for parenteral nutrition are notably deficient in it.

All of these factors point to the importance of some enteral feeding in critically ill patients. Even small amounts such as 5 to 10 mL/hr can be given safely to patients with ileus or intestinal anastomosis, and this small volume is sufficient to minimize intestinal atrophy. If some fat is included with the feeding solution (as is the case with almost all feeding formulas), then the risk of cholestasis is further decreased.

Gastrointestinal Tract Bleeding

Bleeding from the stomach or duodenum is a common problem in critically ill patients and is discussed at this point because the pathogenesis relates in part to the absence of food, buffering, and gastric acid in the stomach. When upper GI bleeding occurs, it is due to ulcerations in the stomach or duodenum and is commonly referred to as *stress ulceration* associated with critical illness. This is a gross misnomer because the ulcerations do not occur in patients because of stress but because of sepsis. It would put the emphasis in the proper place to refer to this as *septic GI bleeding* rather than as *stress GI bleeding* because the most effective prophylaxis is to prevent localized or systemic infection. This is best demonstrated by the experience in burn patients. Upper GI bleeding from gastric or duodenal ulcers was so common in burn patients as to deserve the coining of a specific eponym (Curling's ulcer). In patients treated with older methods of burn surface management, Curling's ulcer was a common occurrence and frequently the cause of death. Now upper GI bleeding is exceptionally rare in burn patients. In my experience in more than 5000 consecutive burn patients in whom a specific protocol was followed and in whom systemic sepsis was very rare, significant upper GI bleeding occurred in only two patients. The prophylactic regimen included gastric feedings and preventing systemic sepsis, but not the administration of H2 blockers.

There is one notable exception to the renaming of ICU GI bleeding as *septic bleeding*. Some patients with brain injury produce huge amounts of gastric acid that can result in the rapid development of the most extensive duodenal ulcers a surgeon will ever encounter. This phenomenon is

TABLE 4-8. Prophylaxis for Upper Gastrointestinal Tract Ulceration and Bleeding and Associated Risks

Treatment	Risk
Therapy to prevent sepsis	None
Optimize $\dot{D}o_2$	Transfusion
Treat anemia	
"Protect" stomach using Carafate (sucralfate)	Nasogastric clamping
Eliminate steroid use	Steroids needed?
Raise gastric pH	Pneumonia
Antacids	Nasogastric clamping
H$_2$ blockers	Cost, patient confusion
Anticholinergic agents	Dry secretions

$\dot{D}o_2$ = oxygen consumption.

referred to as *Cushing's ulcer*. Prophylaxis in this setting depends on the continuous neutralization of the acid.

Although it is commonly said that upper GI ulceration never occurs without acid and pepsin, there is some evidence that gastric ischemia, shock, and some medications such as steroids can predispose critically ill patients to gastric ulceration. Therefore efforts to maintain normal systemic oxygen delivery and normal celiac blood flow and efforts to decrease the use of steroid medications are important aspects of the prophylaxis for GI bleeding. With that done, and with attention focused on preventing sepsis, specific prophylaxis directed toward the stomach and duodenum includes protecting the mucosal barrier of the stomach with a coating agent like Carafate (sucralfate) or maintaining the gastric pH above 4 by buffering or by preventing acid secretion, or both measures. These preventive steps and the risks associated with them are summarized in Table 4-8. If the gastric pH is maintained in the neutral range by antacids, gastric feeding, H$_2$ blockers, or anticholinergic drugs, bacteria and yeast will grow in the stomach because the normal sterilizing effect of gastric acid is neutralized. As a result, the upper and lower intestines become contaminated with greater numbers of different bacteria than are usually present there. In addition the regurgitation of gastric contents with the subsequent aspiration of small amounts of the contents may predispose to the development of nosocomial pneumonia. In most orally intubated patients the risk of serious complications of nosocomial pneumonia is greater than the risk of upper GI bleeding, so that Carafate alone is the best approach to the prophylaxis for GI bleeding. In a very high risk patient, such as one with ongoing sepsis, a history of ulcer disease, or brain injury, additional steps to neutralize the gastric pH are indicated, and the best of these is continuous gastric feeding, if such feeding can be tolerated. Although it is somewhat controversial, the preponderance of evidence indicates that antibiotic treatment to the nasopharynx and stomach in this setting minimizes the risk of nosocomial pneumonia (so-called selective decontamination of the GI tract).

Parenteral Feeding

Commercial preparations for parenteral feeding available in the United States are currently limited to those containing glucose (5% to 45%) and fat (10% to 20%) as the energy sources and amino acid or peptide solutions (2% to 10%) as the protein sources. Both parenteral and tube feedings are planned so that total energy requirements can be met through the fat or carbohydrate contents or both. Any protein administered should be available for anabolic processes. Parenteral feeding with carbohydrate is limited by the sclerotic effect of hyperosmolar solutions on veins, and effective parenteral feeding with carbohydrate alone usually requires that the solutions have a ratio of at least 1 cal/mL (25% sugar). This type of solution must be delivered into an area of rapid blood flow, generally the superior vena cava. Complications still occur, which are discussed later in this chapter. Fat is a more efficient energy source and can be given through peripheral veins in concentrations of either 10% or 20%. The total daily energy requirement can be given as fat or a major portion can be given as fat with the rest as carbohydrate. Both fat and carbohydrate are equally effective sources of energy. The advantage of fat is that it can be administered into peripheral veins; the advantage of carbohydrate is that it costs approximately one tenth the cost of fat. The ratio of the fat to carbohydrate energy sources and the ratio of the total energy sources to grams of protein vary depending on the patient's clinical state. For example, a patient in cardiac failure may require a solution that is low in volume and in sodium but high in calories and protein. A patient with multiple intestinal fistulas may require large volumes, allowing fewer calories and grams of protein per milliliter. Because of the potential problems with central venous cannulation, the administration of 10% glucose, amino acid solutions, and fat through peripheral veins has become popular. Two liters of 10% glucose supply 800 cal, and 500 mL of 20% lipid supply 1000 cal. The total is ample for most patients who are not hypermetabolic.

Any hospital that routinely cares for critically ill patients should have a standardized approach to parenteral nutrition, including the method of vascular access, catheter management, and solution preparation; the makeup of stock solutions; and the protocols for the management of risks and complications. The "standard" solution for total parenteral nutrition is made by mixing equal amounts of 50% glucose and 9% amino acids. This solution contains the equivalent of one carbohydrate calorie per milliliter at a ratio of 25 cal/g of protein. The osmolarity of this solution is 1800 mOsm/L, and it must be given into an area of rapidly flowing blood. The insertion and care of the catheter must be done using a sterile technique. The standard solution can be modified for individual patients by raising or lowering the concentration of glucose and amino acids and by varying the electrolyte and trace metal composition. Vitamins and trace minerals are added to the solution at regular intervals, following the general principle of providing more than the basal requirements, as discussed earlier. The standard solution is supplemented with intravenous fat to provide at least 100 g of fat emulsion each week to prevent fatty acid deficiency. We favor giving 25% to 50% of the calories each day as a fat emulsion. A fat emulsion is usually given through a peripheral vein, although it can be given through a central venous catheter at the same time as the hypertonic glucose solution. Typical formulas are listed in Table 4-9.

The most common complication of total parenteral nutrition is infection on or around the intravascular catheter. Of course, infection can occur with any indwelling vascular catheter, but it is more likely in the presence of hypertonic glucose and protein solutions. If catheter infection is suspected, the catheter must be removed and a new catheter placed. Replacement "over a wire" is sufficient. The second most common complication is hyperglycemia, which can be exacerbated in a septic, insulin-resistant patient. Hyperglycemia is treated with insulin and by the use of fat rather than glucose as the primary calorie source. Other complications are largely those of hyperglycemia, that is, hyperosmolar coma, osmotic diuresis, and localized thrombosis. These complications can be caused by running the solution too rapidly. This is prevented by always using a rate-limiting pump when administering hypertonic solutions. It should be noted that the presence of systemic infection is an indication for nutritional support not a contraindication to placing a central catheter. Other complications are related to disease states and specific amino acids. Aromatic amino acids are neurotransmitter precursors. Symptoms of central nervous system disturbances (confusion, seizures, and coma) occur in patients on a total parenteral nutrition regimen, particularly those with liver dysfunction. These symptoms often cease when the amino acid infusion is stopped. A solution low in aromatic amino acids has been proposed for use in patients with liver failure.

The major trick to the successful clinical use of parenteral nutrition is to develop a precise protocol that covers all steps in the management of this procedure. Many large hospitals have a parenteral nutrition team that supervises the protocol and facilitates the procedure. Where such teams exist, the incidence of complications is minimized, and thus such teams are well worth the expense.

Application of Metabolic Economics to the Critically Ill Patient

Whenever possible, patients who are identified as malnourished through the nutritional assessment process described earlier should be returned to a normal nutritional status before undergoing a major elective operation. Other than this, however, patients who require hospitalization because of critical illness cannot be nutritionally prepared ahead of time. The nutritional status of each patient admitted to the ICU should be evaluated according to the criteria summarized in Table 4-6. Patients who show evidence of

TABLE 4-9. Typical Parenteral Feeding Formulas*

TPN Solution	Carbohydrate (%)	Fat (%)	Protein (%)	mOsm/L	cal/L	Sodium (mEq/L)	Potassium (mEq/L)	Other
10% Glucose	10	0	4.25	880	440	47	23	36 mEq acetate
25% Glucose	25	0	4.25	1825	1020	35	40	25 mEq acetate
10% Lipid	—	10	—	276	1000	0	0	—

*University of Michigan parenteral nutrition team standard solutions. Values given are per liter of solution.
TPN = total parenteral nutrition.

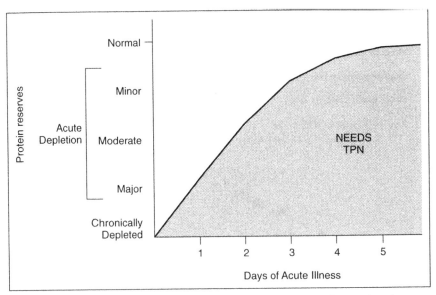

FIGURE 4-11. Guidelines for the timing of the institution of enteral and parenteral feeding in critically ill patients. Most ICU patients fall into the moderate or major acute depletion category and should be started on nutrition the first day or two in the ICU. (TPN = total parenteral nutrition.) (From Bartlett RH. In Dantzker D (ed). Cardiopulmonary Critical Care. New York: Grune & Stratton, 1986.)

malnutrition should be started on a feeding regimen soon after admission. Patients who cannot eat after a few days in the ICU should be started on enteral and parenteral feeding (Figure 4-11).

During the period of the critical illness, nutritional and metabolic status should be assessed daily. Daily measurement of caloric and nitrogen balance is routine in many ICUs. Although the estimates made from tables or graphs vary considerably from the actual protein and caloric requirements, they are better than nothing. The most accurate estimating system is that of Wilmore (Figure 4-4). Fluid balance can be measured accurately in the ICU and the patient should be weighed daily. The correlation of the daily fluid balance with the daily weight is an essential step in evaluating a patient's nutritional status during critical illness. Along with the daily estimation or measurement of the caloric balance, the periodic measurement of acute-phase, protein-dependent reactants such as lymphocytes is also helpful. Many patients reach the state of hypoproteinemia (that is, severe protein malnutrition) while in the critical care unit. However, this should never happen if appropriate attention is given to protein and calorie status. Our algorithm for the management of nutrition in patients with a critical illness is shown in Figure 4-12. We have carried out retrospective studies examining energy balance in critically ill patients with a variety of conditions. In these studies, the survival

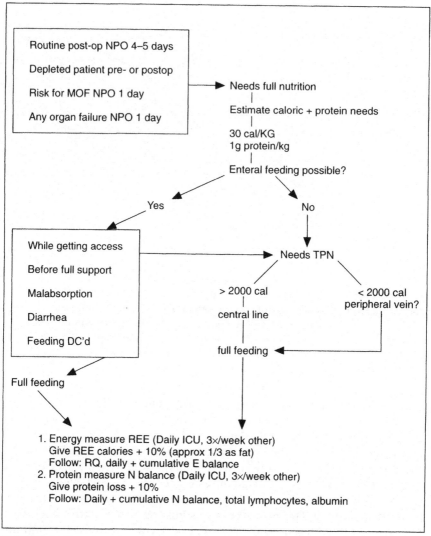

FIGURE 4-12. Nutritional algorithm. (DC'd = discontinued; E = energy; MOF = multiple-organ failure; N = nitrogen; NPO = nothing by mouth; REE = resting energy expenditure; RQ = respiratory quotient; TPN = total parenteral nutrition.)

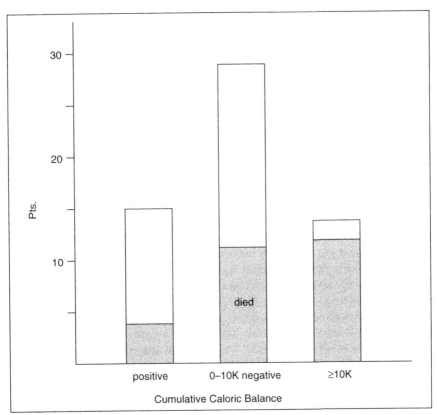

FIGURE 4-13. Outcome in 56 ICU patients with multiple-organ failure correlated with cumulative caloric balance. This is one of the first studies showing that feeding improves survival in ICU patients. (From Bartlett RH, et al. Measurement of metabolism in multiple organ failure. Surgery 1982;92:771–8.)

rate in patients who were in a positive caloric balance at the time of ICU discharge was higher than that in patients in a negative balance. In particular, the mortality was high in patients with a 10,000-cal cumulative deficit at the time of ICU discharge (Figure 4-13). This was true of patients with a variety of illnesses and of specific patient groups with chest trauma and acute renal failure. Furthermore, survival was better when feeding was instituted early in the critical illness. The management of nutrition in patients with acute renal failure is undergoing major changes and is discussed in the next chapter.

Protein and energy nutrition are required in patients in respiratory failure to maintain respiratory muscle strength and bolster the host defenses of the lungs. Patients with pure respiratory failure usually can be fed directly into the GI tract. Energy requirements should be specifically measured in these patients, because overfeeding with carbohydrate results in excess CO_2 production through the conversion of carbohydrate to fat. This positive RQ can

Critical Care Physiology

TABLE 4-10. Nutrition Axioms

1. Estimate or measure caloric and nitrogen balance daily.
2. Use enteral nutrition whenever possible. Even small volumes prevent mucosal atrophy
3. Treat hypoproteinemia with diuresis when appropriate, then with concentrated albumin or plasma.
4. Manage nutrition based on results of balance studies.
5. Absolute lymphocyte count and the prealbumin level are useful markers of acute-phase nutrition, but balance studies are better.
6. Tube feeding–related diarrhea can always be controlled by changing the formula, flora, or fiber.
7. Do not use antacids or H_2 blockers for stress bleeding prophylaxis. The pneumonia risk is higher than the bleeding risk.
8. When gastric pH regulation is used to treat active bleeding, measure the pH regularly and keep it over 4. Many elderly patients are achlorhydric and don't require pH control.

mean that the patient must remain on mechanical ventilation when he or she would otherwise be ready for weaning from the ventilator. Furthermore, overfeeding with carbohydrate is a common cause of ventilator weaning failure, so energy sources should be carefully examined in any patient who has borderline respiratory function.

A patient with system infection (sepsis) has an elevated metabolic rate and an elevated protein catabolic rate. This patient requires an energy and protein supply to meet these needs. The fact that the patient has a systemic infection should not deter the physician from placing a central venous catheter or creating whatever access is required for enteral or parenteral feeding.

The principles in this chapter are summarized in the algorithm given in Figure 4-12 and emphasized in the nutrition axioms given in Table 4-10.

Monographs and Reviews

Berger R, Adams L. Nutritional support in the critical care setting (part I and II). Chest 1989;96:139–150, 372–80.
This review of more than 300 references summarizes the classic and recent literature on this subject.

Bessey PQ. Metabolic response to critical illness. In: Wilmore DW, Brennan MF, Harken AF, Holcroft JW, Meakins JL, eds. Care of the surgical patient: critical care, 2nd ed. New York: Scientific American Medicine, 1994.
An excellent recent review of acute-phase metabolism.

Cerra FB. Hypermetabolism, organ failure, and metabolic support. Surgery 1987;101:1–14.
This paper introduces the concept of repeated insults that occur after initial "priming" as responsible for the pathogenesis of multiple-organ failure.

Cook DJ, Laine LA, Guyatt GH, et al. Nosocomial pneumonia and the role of gastric pH: a meta analysis. Chest 1991;100:7–13.

Tryba M. Sucralfate vs antacids or H2 antagonists for stress ulcer prophylaxis: a meta analysis on efficacy and pneumonia rate. Crit Care Med 1991;19:942–9.

These two "meta analyses" review the same papers and come to opposite conclusions.

Heyland DR, Cook DJ, Guyatt GH. Does the formulation of enteral feeding products influence infectious morbidity and mortality rates in the critically ill patient? A critical review of the evidence. Crit Care Med 1994;22:1192–1202.

This review of the components of enteral feeding preparations includes references to several of the papers showing that luminal glutamine is important to prevent mucosal atrophy.

Kinney JM. Energy requirements of the surgical patients. In: The American College of Surgeons manual, surgical nutrition. Philadelphia: Saunders, 1975.

This review includes a description of the estimated increase in metabolic rate that occurs with various types of critical illness, as discussed in this chapter.

Klieber M. The fire of life. New York: Wiley, 1961.

One of the classic references on nutrition and metabolism. The standard reference for the caloric value of food stuffs, the Weir equation, and a detailed study of metabolism.

Moore FD, Oleson KH, McMurray JD, et al. The body cell mass and its supporting environment. Philadelphia: Saunders, 1963.

The classic monograph summarizing the isotopic dissection of fluid spaces in the body conducted by Moore's laboratory over many years.

Wilmore DW. The metabolic management of the critically ill. New York: Plenum, 1977.

One of the experts in nutrition and metabolism discusses the endocrine and hormonal mediators of metabolism. This book includes a nomogram for predicting metabolic rate in critical illness that is the most accurate predictor, short of actual indirect calorimetry.

Wilmore DW. Catabolic illness. Strategies for enhancing recovery. N Engl J Med 1991;325:695–703.

This review includes an analysis of the cytokine and hormonal mediators of the stress response, specific nutrient fluids, and growth factors, including the author's extensive experience with growth hormones.

Selected Reports

AMA Department of Foods and Nutrition. Guidelines for essential trace element preparations for parenteral use: a statement of an expert panel. JAMA 1979;241:2050–4.

The recommended dosages given in this chapter are based on this publication.

Bartlett RH, Allyn PA, Medley T, Wetmore N. Nutritional therapy based on positive caloric balance in burn patients. Arch Surg 1977;112:974.

One of the first studies demonstrating the value of managing nutrition based on indirect calorimetry findings in critically ill patients.

Bartlett RH, Dechert RE, Mault J, Ferguson S, Kaiser AM, Erlandson EE. Measurement of metabolism in multiple organ failure. Surgery 1982;92:771–8.

The first study that correlated a positive cumulative caloric balance with survival in critically ill patients.

Bower RH, Muggia-Sullam M, Vallgren S, et al. Branched chain amino acid–enriched solutions in the septic patient. A randomized prospective trial. Ann Surg 1986;203:13–20.

Many modifications of parenteral feeding formulations have been studied in animals and few have been found to have an impact on clinical outcome in patients. This randomized study of branched-chain amino acid–enriched solutions showed no improvement compared with the outcome in patients who received conventional parenteral solutions.

Cahill G. Starvation in man. N Engl J Med 1970;282:668–75.

A classic reference on the effects of starvation and starvation adaptation in normal human subjects.

Christou NV, MacLean APH, Meakins JL. Host defense in blunt trauma: interrelationships of kinetics of anergy and depressed neutrophil function. Nutritional status in sepsis. J Trauma 1980;28:833–41.

One of several papers published by the Montreal group relating the immune response measured by skin test reactivity in critically ill patients to malnutrition.

Dechert RE, Cerny JC, Bartlett RH. Measurement of elemental nitrogen by chemiluminescence: an evaluation of the Antek nitrogen analyzer system. JPEN 1990;14:195–7.

Description of the development of a device for protein balance measurements in the ICU.

Driks MR, Craven DE, Celli BR. Nosocomial pneumonia in intubated patients given sucralfate as compared with antacids or H2 blockers: the role of gastric colonization. N Engl J Med 1987;317:1376–82.

One of the first studies to demonstrate pneumonia associated with gastric bacterial overgrowth in the pH-neutral stomach.

Dudrick SJ, Wilmore DW, Vars HM, Rhoades JE. Can intravenous feeding as a sole means of nutrition support growth in the child and restore weight loss in an adult? An affirmative answer. Ann Surg 1969;169:974–90.

This is the classic paper first describing successful total parenteral nutrition in detail.

Gazzaniga AB, Bartlett RH, Shobe JB. Nitrogen balance in patients receiving either fat or carbohydrate for total intravenous nutrition. Ann Surg 1975;182:163–8.

This is one of the first papers to show that fat can be used as the sole energy source in parenteral nutrition.

Harris JA, Benedict FG. Biometric studies of basal metabolism in man. Washington, DC: Carnegie Institute of Washington, Publication #269, 1919.

The original publication on the typical oxygen consumption and basal metabolic rate in normal volunteers.

Kresowik TF, Dechert RE, Mault JR, Arnoldi DK, Whitehouse WM Jr, Bartlett RH. Does nutritional support affect survival in critically ill patients? Surg Forum 1984;35:108–11.

Patients who achieved a positive caloric balance early in the course of their stay in the ICU had better survival than did patients fed in a conventional fashion.

Moore FA, Moore EE, Kudsk KA, et al. Clinical benefits of an immune-enhancing diet for early postinjury enteral feeding. J Trauma 1994;37:607–15.

The incidence of organ failure was found to be less in trauma patients fed an enteral diet high in protein, glutamine, and branched-chain amino acids than it was in patients on a conventional tube feeding regimen.

Sargent J, Gotch F, Borah M, et al. Urea kinetics: a guide to nutritional management of acute renal failure. Am J Clin Nutr 1978;31:1696–1702.

This classic paper describes the method to define protein and urea kinetics in anuric and oliguric patients.

Shizgal HM, Milne CA, Spanier AH. The effect of nitrogen-sparing, intravenously administered fluids on postoperative body composition. Surgery 1979;85:496–503.

This study showed that any source of protein can cause an increase in the body cell mass in postoperative patients.

van der Hulst RRWJ, vanKreel BK, von Meyenfeldt MF, et al. Glutamine and the preservation of gut integrity. Lancet 1993;341:1363–70.

One of many studies showing that luminal glutamine prevents mucosal atrophy in patients being fed parenterally or enterally.

Weissman C, Askanazi J, Forse RA, et al. The metabolic and ventilatory response to the infusion of stress hormones. Ann Surg 1986;203:408–12.

One of the classic papers describing the induction of the hypermetabolic protein catabolic state in normal persons in response to the infusion of stress-related hormones.

5

Renal Physiology and Pathophysiology

Renal physiology is simplified and summarized in Figure 5-1. Blood perfuses the renal cortex and extracellular fluid (ECF) is filtered through the glomeruli at a rate of approximately 7 L/hr. Almost all (99.4%) of this fluid is resorbed in the proximal and distal tubules, leaving approximately 40 mL/hr to run down the ureters into the urinary bladder. The only purpose of the overdesign of this system is to excrete the by-products of protein metabolism and a few other molecules that cannot be excreted through the lungs or liver. If only 25% of the nephrons are working, blood electrolyte and urea levels can still be maintained in the normal range. If only 10% of the nephrons are working, azotemia occurs but life goes on. If less than 5% of the nephrons are working, fatal uremia or congestive heart failure occurs unless some type of mechanical renal replacement therapy is implemented.

Usually nephrons fail altogether, although there are situations in which specific nephron functions are lost preferentially. The most common of these is polyuric or nonoliguric renal failure in which glomerular filtrate is produced but the proximal tubular handling of sodium, potassium, and urea is abnormal. In this setting, the patient may excrete adequate or even very large amounts of urine that is of poor quality—high in sodium, low in potassium, and low in urea.

Renal function is most commonly evaluated by simply measuring the amount of urea or creatinine in serum or urine. If these measurements are abnormal, renal function can be more specifically characterized by calculating the creatinine clearance or the fractional excretion of sodium or urea. The definitions of and formulas for making these measurements are listed in Table 5-1.

In the intensive care unit (ICU) renal function is taken for granted and is counted on to offset the gross excesses in the quantities of salt and fluid administered to patients. All manner of fluid, electrolyte, and metabolic

5. Renal Physiology and Pathophysiology

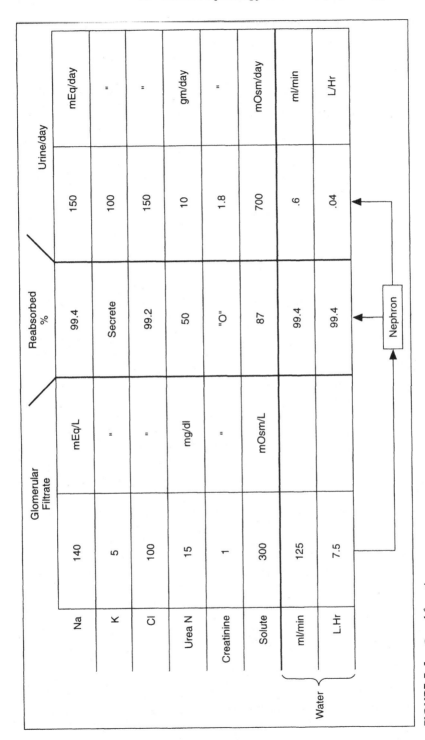

FIGURE 5-1. Renal function.

TABLE 5-1. Definitions of Renal Function Variables and Formulas for Determining

Abbreviation	Definition	Equation	Normal Value
GFR	Glomerular filtration rate	—	2 mL/kg/min
Osm	Osmolarity/liter	—	urine = 300–1300 mOsm/L; ECF = 300 mOsm/L
CrCl	Creatinine clearance	$\dfrac{U_{creat} \times V}{P_{creat}}$	100 mL/min
$F_E Na$	Fractional excretion of sodium	$\dfrac{U_{Na} \times P_{creat}}{P_{Na} \times U_{creat}}$	< 1%
$F_E Urea$	Fractional excretion of urea	$\dfrac{U_{urea} \times P_{creat}}{P_{urea} \times U_{creat}}$	> 50%

creat = creatinine; ECF = extracellular fluid; P = plasma concentration; U = urine concentration.

disorders are automatically rectified by normal renal function. We take advantage of this in patients to clear drugs, salt, and metabolites that are often given in excess. In fact, kidney physiology comes to our attention only when function fails. Consequently the rest of this discussion is focused on the causes, pathophysiologic consequences, and treatment of renal failure.

Acute renal failure (ARF) is defined as an abrupt decrease in kidney function that results in the accumulation of nitrogenous solutes. Urine output in ARF may be oliguric (urine output of less than 400 mL/day) or nonoliguric (urine output is normal or increased but solute clearance is markedly decreased). The mortality associated with ARF in critically ill patients is high (50% to 90%) because ARF is usually just one component of severe multiple-organ failure. The mortality associated with nonoliguric ARF is significantly less than that associated with oliguric ARF, although many patients become oliguric and suffer the resulting poor outcome. Regardless of the urine output, the sequelae of ARF result from the retention of metabolic wastes, as shown by a progressive rise in the blood urea nitrogen (BUN) and serum creatinine concentrations. Hypervolemia and electrolyte imbalances further complicate the management of oliguric ARF.

ARF is commonly classified according to whether it is caused by prerenal, postrenal, or intrinsic parenchymal disease. The discussion in this chapter is limited to parenchymal disease.

Parenchymal Disease

Parenchymal abnormalities include acute tubular necrosis (ATN) and pigment nephropathy (resulting from circulating myoglobin and hemoglobin) as well as the disorders produced by nephrotoxic agents (various drugs and contrast material). Other causes of parenchymal disease such as acute glomerular nephritis and vasculitis are not typically responsible for ARF in the ICU patient and are not discussed in this chapter.

Acute Tubular Necrosis

ATN results from ischemia in the renal parenchyma and is the most common pathologic finding noted in ARF. Under conditions of diminishing renal blood flow, perfusion of the kidneys is first maintained by vasomotor responses, which cause the afferent arterioles to dilate and the efferent arterioles to constrict. As continued hypotension is detected by the juxtaglomerular apparatus, the renin-angiotensin system is activated in concert with the sympathetic release of other vasoactive hormones. These substances cause the afferent arterioles to constrict, and this further exacerbates the cortical hypoperfusion. As a result, the glomerular filtration rate is sharply reduced and the tubules experience profound ischemia. With damage to the tubular system, casts of cellular debris obstruct the lumen and cellular edema ensues. As tubular cells necrose and slough off, glomerular ultrafiltrate leaks back across the proximal tubular membrane into the interstitium. It has recently been suggested that this "back-leakage" of luminal fluid into the peritubular space causes vascular congestion within the renal parenchyma and may contribute to the prolongation of ARF. The absence of these glomerular changes in the presence of adequate cortical blood flow may account for the maintenance of urine output that occurs in nonoliguric ARF and the recovery phase of oliguric ARF. Thus, ATN represents a spectrum of cortical ischemic injury, ranging from polyuria with tubular dysfunction, to temporary anuria, to renal cortical necrosis with chronic anuria.

Pigment Nephropathy

Pigment nephropathy is a common cause of ARF and may occur as a consequence of trauma, burns, operation, or a hemodynamic catastrophe. With the occurrence of ischemia or blunt injury affecting large muscle masses, myoglobin is released into the circulation. In the kidney it is filtered from blood and resorbed by the tubule. Although myoglobin is not a direct nephrotoxin, in the presence of aciduria it is converted to ferrihemate, which is toxic to renal cells. Rhabdomyolysis should be suspected in patients suffering from burns, trauma, seizures, alcohol or drug intoxication, prolonged ischemia to muscle groups, and extended coma. Diagnosis can be made on the basis of an elevated creatine phosphokinase activity and a urine microscopy study that shows a prominent amount of heme pigment without red blood cells in the urine sediment. Hyperkalemia and an elevated serum creatinine level are also findings consistent with injury to muscle masses. Prevention of myoglobin-induced ARF may include the administration of diuretics and the alkalization of urine, although the efficacy of this therapy has yet to be determined. The prophylactic infusion of haptoglobin is also being tested as a means of preventing ARF in burn patients.

Nephrotoxic Agents

Drug-induced ARF is responsible for approximately 20% of all cases of ARF. Its pathophysiology differs according to the offending agent. Through the normal processes of resorption and secretion, the kidney is exposed to high concentrations of drugs and solutes, which may be toxic. This problem is compounded by hypovolemia, which causes the increased resorption of water and solutes and exposes the lumen to even higher concentrations of toxins. Although the damage to tubular function can be significant, much drug-induced ARF remains nonoliguric owing to the sparing of glomerular function.

Radiographic contrast dye has been documented to cause ARF. The incidence of contrast nephropathy is approximately 1% to 10%, and the likelihood of its developing in a particular patient can be predicted by the presence of a number of various risk factors. These include the contrast load, patient age, and the presence of preexisting renal insufficiency or diabetes, although the validity of some of these factors is currently disputed. The incidence of contrast nephropathy in patients with normal renal function is significantly lower, at 1% to 2%. Contrast nephropathy is usually experienced as an asymptomatic, transient rise in the creatinine level, but oliguric renal failure requiring hemodialysis may eventuate. Induced diuresis with fluids and diuretics before contrast injection may cause the incidence and severity of ARF in high-risk patients to be decreased.

Management of ARF

ARF rarely occurs in an isolated fashion in critically ill patients. Rather it is only one component of a multiple-organ failure syndrome that is often accompanied by infection. Management of these patients should therefore be focused on treatment of the underlying disease process, or processes. The development of ARF complicates the care of ICU patients by introducing difficulties in fluid, electrolyte, and nutritional management. The adverse effects of renal replacement therapies further compound these problems. A favorable outcome can be accomplished only through aggressive intervention. This includes surgical drainage of a septic focus, excision of necrotic tissue, early implementation of effective renal replacement therapy, and full nutritional support.

General Care of Patients with ARF

Our algorithm for the evaluation and management of ARF is shown in Figure 5-2. The treatment of patients with nonoliguric ARF may differ little from that required for identical patients with normal renal function. Management of fluids, solutes, and nutrition is usually unaffected by nonoliguric ARF, although the BUN level may be elevated. The extent of renal dysfunction is limited and almost always reversible. Renal replacement therapies, with their inherent complications, are rarely necessary.

Oliguria and anuria pose several management difficulties. In the absence of normal urine output, problems of fluid overload can lead to anasarca, pulmonary edema, and congestive heart failure. The pharmacokinetics of drugs becomes difficult to predict as a result of the decreased elimination and increased volume of distribution. In light of these risks, the volume status of patients with ARF must be monitored carefully. Fluid intake and output must be tabulated precisely, and body weight should be measured daily. Pulmonary artery catheterization may be necessary to monitor more closely the hemodynamic status of these patients. Treatment options for hypervolemia consist of fluid restriction or fluid removal using artificial kidney techniques. However, fluid restriction limits the amount of intravenous medications that can be administered and may preclude adequate nutrition.

ARF can create severe derangements in the electrolyte and acid-base balance. Serum electrolyte levels should be measured daily. Of all the electrolyte abnormalities that might occur with ARF, hyperkalemia is the most serious. Under the conditions of hypercatabolism and tissue necrosis that arise in these patients, large amounts of potassium may be generated and may accumulate over a short time. Acute hyperkalemia decreases cardiac excitability, which may ultimately result in asystole. These events are usually preceded by changes in the electrocardiogram that indicate the presence of hyperkalemia. These changes include loss of P waves, widening of the QRS complex, and peaked T waves. Immediate treatment of hyperkalemia consists of the infusion of glucose-insulin, calcium gluconate, and bicarbonate. However, these measures can bring about only transient shifts in the potassium from extracellular to intracellular spaces and are of limited value. Removal of potassium must be accomplished with renal replacement therapy or the administration of ion-exchange resins. Other electrolyte abnormalities such as hyponatremia, hyperphosphatemia, hypocalcemia, and metabolic acidosis are common with ARF and must be monitored closely. Their treatment consists of appropriate additions or restrictions of intravenous solutions and effective use of the artificial kidney.

Although poorly understood, platelet dysfunction and coagulopathy are often associated with ARF. A reproducible platelet defect can be demonstrated experimentally with a BUN of 100 mg/dL. However, the cause of this defect has yet to be identified.

140 Critical Care Physiology

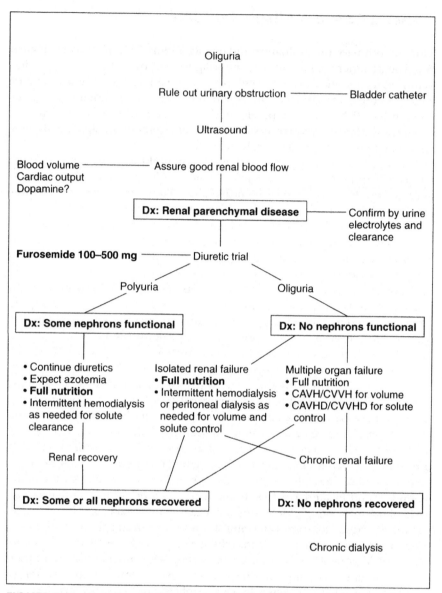

FIGURE 5-2. Acute renal failure management algorithm. (CAVH = continuous arteriovenous hemofiltration; CAVHD = continuous arteriovenous hemodiafiltration; CVVH = continuous venovenous hemofiltration; CVVHD = continuous venovenous hemodiafiltration; PD = peritoneal dialysis.)

Anemia also accompanies ARF in the surgical patient. In addition to the blood loss resulting from hemorrhage or operation, erythropoietin production has been shown to decrease in these patients in direct proportion to decreasing renal function.

Nutrition and ARF

The goal of nutritional support in patients with ARF is to provide optimal amounts of calorie and protein substrates to minimize autocatabolism and promote tissue anabolism, wound healing, and sustained immune function. In any discussion of nutrition and renal failure, it is necessary to point out the distinction between acute and chronic renal failure. Patients in chronic renal failure are generally healthy and have energy requirements that differ little from those of patients with normal function. Protein intake is required only for metabolic turnover and is restricted to minimize the production of urea and other products of protein metabolism.

By contrast, the metabolic requirements of a patient with ARF are those of a critically ill, hospitalized patient. Actual measurement of the resting energy expenditure has shown that the caloric requirements of patients with multiple-organ failure suffering from ARF average 50% more than those of normal, healthy persons. Measured protein requirements are also increased to as much as 2.5 g/kg to promote anabolic wound healing and ensure sustained immune function. For these patients, protein restriction is counterproductive and potentially detrimental. Urea generation is best minimized by giving the patients enough energy substrates (carbohydrates and lipids) to prevent the cannibalization of endogenous protein as an energy source. In recent years investigations of measures that emphasize energy and protein balance have shown they lead to an improved outcome from ARF.

A positive energy balance may also make the management of uremia and hyperkalemia less difficult. When a patient receives fewer calories than those expended, the difference must be made up for from endogenous stores. In a well-nourished person, the carbohydrate stores rarely exceeds 2500 k cal. After this has been depleted, lipid and protein stores are mobilized. In the diseased state, endogenous protein is preferentially catabolized as an energy substrate in the absence of readily available glucose. With the catabolism of protein, urea is generated. In addition, the catabolic wasting of tissues and cells liberates excess potassium. Maintenance of positive energy balance with glucose and lipids should reduce protein catabolism, urea generation, and hyperkalemia. Our group has shown that survival in patients with ARF correlates with a positive caloric balance (Figure 5-3).

Although protein restriction may be advocated in patients with chronic renal failure, the protein requirements in those with ARF are usually elevated. Abel and colleagues were among the first to suggest that survival is

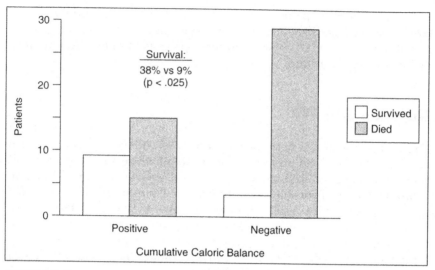

FIGURE 5-3. Survival and nutrition in acute renal failure. Patients in oliguric renal failure had better outcome when positive caloric balance was achieved. (From Mault JR, Bartlett RH. Acute renal failure. In: Greenfield LJ, ed. Complications in surgery and trauma. Philadelphia: Lippincott, 1989: 149–62.)

improved in patients with ARF when amino acids are added to the intravenous nutrition. Others have confirmed these findings. The two important concerns regarding protein supplementation in ARF are what type of protein and how much to administer. The rate of protein catabolism revealed by various studies ranges from 70 to 200 g/day. In light of this wide range, actual measurement of the protein balance is desirable. The protein catabolic rate of an oliguric patient can be reasonably approximated by calculating the urea generation rate. In this calculation, changes in the BUN level and fluid balance are recorded for a 24-hour period. The nitrogen content is also determined from collections of dialysate or ultrafiltrate, from nasogastric suction material, wound drain material, and the like, obtained over the same time interval. Assuming that the urea produced by protein catabolism is not reused and that it is contained within the extracellular space, the urea generation rate can be calculated. With this information the daily protein balance can be monitored. Maintenance of a positive protein balance is the goal, although this may be difficult to achieve. Most investigators have supplemented protein at a rate of 0.5 to 1.0 g/kg/day, and the effects of providing larger amounts have yet to be studied.

Much effort has been devoted to determining the optimum types of proteins and amino acids to administer to patients with ARF. Abel and associates concluded that a solution consisting of only essential amino acids should be given, but subsequent studies have shown that full protein feeding with essential and nonessential amino acids is the important factor.

The current recommendations regarding nutrition in patients with ARF are as follows:

1. To minimize protein catabolism, glucose and lipids should be supplied to maintain a positive energy balance.
2. Protein should be administered with the goal of achieving a positive nitrogen balance.
3. In the absence of conclusive evidence supporting the use of specialized formulations (that is, essential or branched-chain amino acid solutions), use of a mixed amino acid solution is recommended.
4. Daily measurement of protein and energy balance is the best way to plan nutritional therapy.

Renal Replacement Therapy

With the first use of hemodialysis by Kolff in 1944, the reversible nature of ARF was recognized. Since that time, hemodialysis has become the standard treatment for keeping patients alive who would otherwise die from kidney disease.

Indications for the use of renal replacement therapy include fluid overload (pulmonary edema and congestive heart failure), hyperkalemia, metabolic acidosis, uremic encephalopathy, coagulopathy, and acute poisoning. Three modes of renal replacement therapy are currently available for the treatment of ARF. The features of each of these therapies are contrasted in Table 5-2 and described in the following sections.

Modes of Renal Replacement Therapy

Hemodialysis

Hemodialysis has been used extensively over the past four decades to manage both acute and chronic renal failure. In the contemporary form of hemodialysis, blood is circulated through a porous hollow-fiber or cellulose membrane that is permeable to solutes of less than 2000 daltons. An isotonic solution surrounds the membrane that provides a concentration gradient for the selective removal of solutes such as potassium, urea, and creatinine while maintaining plasma concentrations of sodium, chloride, and bicarbonate. A roller pump is used to maintain an extracorporeal blood flow of approximately 300 mL/min by means of an arteriovenous shunt or a double-lumen venovenous access. The transmembrane pressure gradient created by the pump affects the amount of fluid removed. Systemic or regional anticoagulation is required for this procedure, although less heparin may be used in patients with a baseline coagulopathy. Hemodialysis is typically performed every other day for a 3- to 4-hour period but is required more frequently in catabolic patients with a high urea generation rate. The solute

TABLE 5-2. Comparison of Renal Replacement Therapies

Variable	Hemodialysis	Peritoneal dialysis	CAVH/CAVHD
Description	Rapid, intermittent	Slow, intermittent	Slow, continuous
Access	Arteriovenous or venovenous	Abdominal catheter	Arteriovenous or venovenous
Anticoagulation	Required	None required	Required
Solute removal	Excellent	Excellent	Good with standard CAVH; excellent with CAVHD
Fluid removal	Good to excellent	Good	Excellent
Hemodynamic instability	Significant	None	None
Risks of procedure	Hypotension/hypoxemia; hemorrhage; dysequilibrium syndrome	Infection/peritonitis; intraabdominal adhesions; respiratory distress	Dehydration: hemorrhage; electrolyte imbalance
Overall appraisal	Useful for urgent removal of solutes or poisons; hemodynamic instability limits use in intensive care patients	Contraindicated with abdominal operation; useful in burn patients and poor vascular access	Allows great flexibility with fluid and electrolyte balance; solute removal enhanced with CAVHD

CAVH = continuous arteriovenous hemofiltration; CAVHD = continuous arteriovenous hemodialysis.
From: Mault JR, Bartlett RH. Acute renal failure. In: Greenfield LJ, ed. Complications in surgery and trauma. Philadelphia: Lippincott, 1989.

and volume removal accomplished by hemodialysis are very efficient relative to the removal achieved by other methods of renal replacement. This property is reflected in the clearance of water-soluble drugs such as aminoglycoside, cephalosporins, and penicillins. Plasma concentrations may be decreased by as much as 50% per treatment; accordingly, these drugs should be administered on a posttreatment schedule and the serum concentration should be monitored more closely. Hemodialysis is also the method of choice for the rapid removal of life-threatening toxins and poisons.

Although the incidence of complications from hemodialysis is insignificant in patients with chronic renal failure, frequent and often profound complications may occur in critically ill patients with ARF. In the acute setting, hemodialysis has been shown to cause hypotension, hypoxemia, and hemolysis and to precipitate cardiac arrhythmias. These events limit the application of dialysis in patients in an unstable condition. The major source of these complications is an acute increase in the metabolic rate (oxygen consumption), presumably caused by the activation of white blood cells contacting the dialyzer. If the patient cannot mount an increase in oxygen delivery, the ratio will fall below 2 and shock will ensue.

Peritoneal Dialysis

Peritoneal dialysis is performed by the infusion of several liters of a sterile electrolyte solution along with hypertonic glucose into the abdominal space. Using the peritoneal membrane as a selective barrier, the dialysate solution creates an osmotic pressure gradient that extracts ECF and solutes out of the mesenteric circulation and into the peritoneal cavity, which is then drained after an equilibration period of 1 to 2 hours. The rate of extracellular volume removal usually ranges from 0.5 to 1.0 L/hr, although greater fluid and solute clearance can be accomplished by using larger volumes of dialysate and performing exchange cycles more frequently. Use of an automated delivery system makes this a relatively simple procedure with respect to nursing time and training.

Peritoneal dialysis has several advantages over other methods of renal substitution. It does not require vascular access or systemic anticoagulation, making it useful in patients with peripheral vascular disease or with a heightened risk of hemorrhage. In addition, the slow rate of equilibration and fluid extraction minimizes the problems of dysequilibrium and hemodynamic compromise that arise with conventional hemodialysis.

However, peritoneal dialysis is associated with many risks and complications, particularly in surgical patients. The most frequent and serious of these complications is catheter infection and peritonitis. Rigid peritoneal catheters inserted percutaneously in the acute setting become predictably colonized after 48 to 72 hours. Subcutaneously placed silicone elastomer catheters are associated with a lower incidence of peritonitis (1.6 episodes per patient-year) and should be implanted for the prolonged use necessary for peritoneal dialysis. Other access-related complications include visceral injury at the time of catheter placement and the formation of intraabdominal adhesions. In light of these risks, peritoneal dialysis is generally the last-choice method of renal replacement in patients who have undergone abdominal operation or sustained trauma.

Other complications of peritoneal dialysis include hyperglycemia secondary to the hypertonic glucose in the dialysate and respiratory distress resulting from the reduced diaphragmatic compliance stemming from the increased intraabdominal pressure. Finally, repeated lavage of the peritoneal cavity causes a protein (not urea) loss of 10 g/day or greater and may exacerbate malnutrition in patients with catabolic ARF.

Continuous Arteriovenous Hemofiltration

Continuous arteriovenous hemofiltration (CAVH) was conceived by Kramer and colleagues in 1977 and is specifically intended for the treatment of ARF. CAVH is an extracorporeal ultrafiltration technique that removes ECF across a synthetic membrane propelled by the hydrostatic pressure gradient created between indwelling arterial and venous catheters. With a systolic blood pressure of 80 mm Hg or greater, blood flows through the porous hollow-fiber capillary membrane at a rate of 50 to 150 mL/min, thus driving plasma water and solutes of up to 10,000 daltons out of the hemofilter at 500 to 700 mL/hr. A replacement solution formulated to resemble ECF without the toxic solutes is infused simultaneously into the venous access of the circuit at a rate appropriate to achieve a desired hourly fluid balance. This exchange transfusion of 12 to 17 liters of ECF per day provides a clearance of approximately 10 to 14 g of urea per day (assuming a BUN concentration of 80 mg/dL). The mechanics of CAVH are illustrated in Figure 5-4. Arteriovenous access is accomplished by the percutaneous cannulation of the femoral artery and veins, and this is associated with a low incidence of complications. Although full systemic anticoagulation is not necessary for CAVH, heparinization of the extracorporeal circuit is required, usually at a rate of 500 units/hr. CAVH is run continuously for as many days as renal replacement is required. Hemofilter performance (as monitored by the ultrafiltration rate) decreases over time, requiring replacement with a new hemofilter approximately every 2 days.

Experience with CAVH in the treatment of critically ill ARF patients in unstable condition has revealed little or no incidence of hemodynamic instability. The stable nature of this therapy is attributed to its slow and continuous fluid and solute removal and to the fact that the membrane (polysulfone) does not induce complement activation when in contact with blood.

With ultrafiltration rates averaging 10 to 12 L/day, CAVH also permits great flexibility in the volume management and eliminates the need for fluid restriction in patients with oliguric ARF. Fluid balance and serum electrolyte concentrations can be titrated to any value in a matter of hours by manipulating the composition and rate of the replacement solution. CAVH facilitates the provision of optimal amounts of nutrition to patients with ARF. A typical example is shown in Figure 5-5.

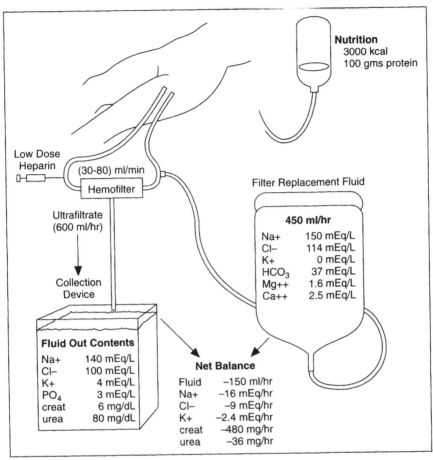

FIGURE 5-4. Principles of management of continuous arteriovenous hemofiltration. (From: Mault JR, et al. Continuous arteriovenous filtration: an effective treatment for surgical acute renal failure. Surgery 1987;101:478–84.)

Continuous Venovenous Hemofiltration

If arterial access is a problem, continuous hemofiltration can be carried out by actively withdrawing venous blood with the pump, then pumping the blood through a hemofilter and returning it to the venous system. This is commonly done with a double-lumen catheter. This technique is commonly used in preference to CAVH because it eliminates the need for access into the femoral or brachial artery. However, it does invite the complications associated with a mechanical pump, and the risks of hemolysis and air embolism are heightened. The principles of managing fluid balance in patients undergoing continuous venovenous hemofiltration (CVVH) are exactly the same as those in patients being treated with CAVH.

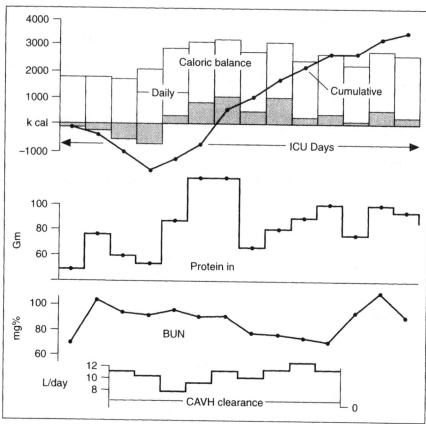

FIGURE 5-5. Oliguric renal failure and a rectoperitoneal abscess developed in a 24-year-old man after he underwent renal and pancreatic transplantation. Continuous arteriovenous hemofiltration (CAVH) was started when his BUN level rose to 100/dL. With CAVH at a rate of 10 L/day, uremia is controlled and protein/caloric feeding is given, resulting in resolution of the abscess and eventual recovery.

Continuous Hemodiafiltration

Solute clearance with CAVH or CVVH is limited by the ultrafiltration and replacement fluid exchange rate. In patients whose urea generation rate is high, the solute removal achieved by continuous hemofiltration may be inadequate and variations of the technique may be used to enhance clearance. The best of these variations is continuous arteriovenous or venovenous hemodiafiltration. In continuous hemodiafiltration, the same filter and circuit as those used in continuous hemofiltration are used but a dialysate bath is also employed to augment solute clearance. The principle of this approach is that small-molecule solutes will pass from blood to the filtrate by direct filtration as well as by convection in response to a concentration gradient. In

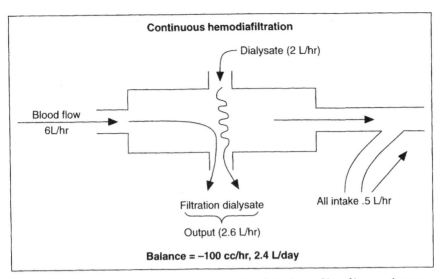

FIGURE 5-6. Adding dialysate to the outside of the hemofilter fibers enhances solute clearance. In this example, dialysate runs through at a rate of 2 L/hr.

straightforward continuous hemofiltration the concentration of urea and potassium is the same outside the hemofilter tubule as it is in the blood. By rapidly diluting the filtrate with a dialysate solution that does not contain urea or potassium, some of these molecules are removed by convection as blood passes through the hemofilter, just as they are normally cleared during conventional hemodialysis. By adding dialysate to the filtration side of the filter, small molecule clearance can be enhanced by a factor of 3 or 4, thereby increasing clearances associated with an increasing rate of dialysate flow. Because the filtration rate is about 600 mL/min, dialysate must run through quite rapidly for any significant dilution and improved solute clearance to occur. This process is usually limited by the simple mechanical problems of hanging and discarding bags or bottles of fluid in the ICU. We typically run dialysate at a rate of 2 or 3 L/hr on a continuous basis. A different and perhaps more efficient method is to run through 30 or 40 liters of dialysate over the course of an hour or so once or twice a day. The principles involved in continuous hemodiafiltration are illustrated in Figure 5-6.

Slow Continuous Ultrafiltration

Sometimes it is desirable to institute continuous hemofiltration to rapidly remove salt and water from a patient who is not in renal failure. Because it is not necessary to achieve the clearance of potassium, urea, or other solutes in this setting, it is not necessary to design a filtration replacement fluid or a continuous dialysis system for this purpose. Instead ECF is simply filtered out of the flowing blood at the rate of 200 to 400 mL/hr without specific replacement. This approach is commonly called *slow continuous ultrafiltration* (SCUF). SCUF is customarily used in critically ill patients with intravenous fluids running in at the rate of 100 to 200 mL/hr and urine coming out at a similar rate. Therefore with SCUF it is possible to achieve a net hourly loss of 100 to 400 mL of ECF per hour. The fluid removed is isotonic. If hypovolemia occurs, the ECF is replaced with packed cells or concentrated protein solutions, while the net negative hourly output is maintained. It should be noted that, in the absence of specific replacement fluid, this will result in a significant loss of bicarbonate over a period of hours and metabolic acidosis will ensue.

Guidelines for Renal Replacement Therapy in ARF

The current recommendations for renal replacement therapy in patients with ARF are as follows:

1. Volume (intravenous fluids, total parenteral nutrition, and so on) should be provided as needed for the patient, independent of the method of renal replacement.
2. Renal replacement therapy should be instituted early in ARF, before hypervolemia, azotemia, or hyperkalemia occurs.
3. For severely ill patients with ARF, CAVH or CVVH is the renal replacement therapy of choice (as opposed to hemodialysis or peritoneal dialysis).
4. If solute clearance is insufficient with continuous hemofiltration, convert to continuous hemodiafiltration or supplement it with standard hemodialysis.
5. Peritoneal dialysis may be used when vascular access is unavailable or the risk of hemorrhage is prohibitive.
6. Hemodynamically stable patients with isolated ARF should be treated with intermittent hemodialysis or peritoneal dialysis.

Prognosis

The survival of patients with ARF is a function of the successful treatment of the primary disease from which the renal failure was derived. The anephric patient supported with renal replacement therapy survives until disease of some other organ system supervenes. In a study of patients with "pure" ATN after renal transplantation, Mentzer and colleagues found the mortality associated with ischemic ATN in the absence of other organ failure was 6%. By contrast, the mortality associated with multiple-organ failure complicated by ARF ranges from 50% to 90%.

Investigation of the conditions associated with ARF has identified several prognostic indicators. In a group of 65 patients with postoperative ARF, Cioffi and colleagues found a significant difference between 12 survivors and 53 nonsurvivors ($p < 0.05$) in the number of organ systems failed, the

5. Renal Physiology and Pathophysiology

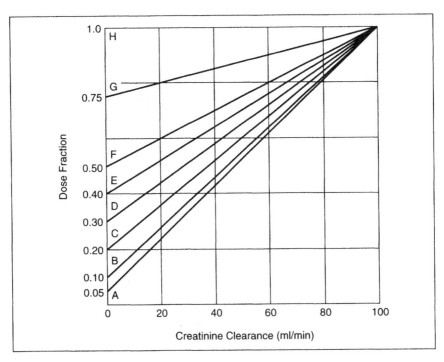

Drug Dosage in Renal Failure

1. Give usual loading dose
2. Measure or estimate creatinine clearance (C_{creat}).
3. Look up dosing line (A–H) for chosen antibiotic: e.g., gentamicin is line A.
4. Read dose fraction from graph at that C_{creat}.
5. Dose fraction times dose for patients with normal renal function per 24 hours equals maintenance dose per 24 hours.
6. Choose dosing interval you deem appropriate.
7. Additional doses may be required if patient needs hemodialysis.

Acyclovir, B
Amikacin, A
Amphotericin-B, G
Ampicillin, B
Carbenicillin, B
Cefamandole, B
Cefazolin, A
Cefotaxime, D
Cefotixin, A
Cephalexin, A
Cephalothin, A
Chloramphenicol, G

Clindamycin, G
Cloxacillin, F
Colistimethate, B
Dicloxacillin, E
Doxycycline, H
Erythromycin, D
Gentamicin, A
Ketoconazole, H
Methicillin, B
Metronidazole, G
Moxalactam, B

Nafcillin, D
Oxacillin, F
Penicillin-G, B
Piperacillin, D
Streptomycin, A
Sulfamethoxazole, E
Sulfisoxazole, F
Ticarcillin, B
Tobramycin, A
Trimethoprim, F
Vancomycin, A

FIGURE 5-7. Adjusting drug dosage based on creatine clearance.
(Adapted from: Clin Nephrol 1977;7:81.)

interval from the onset of ARF to the first dialysis session, the maximum serum creatinine level before dialysis, and the presence of cardiac failure. Corwin and colleagues noted similar indicators in a group of 151 patients with ARF and also that 90% of deaths were due to sepsis or multiple-organ failure. Both survival and recovery of renal function were significantly better in patients with nonoliguric as opposed to oliguric ARF.

In patients who survive the acute phase of illness, recovery of renal function after ARF is dependent on the type and extent of injury to the renal parenchyma. Renal replacement therapy may be required for several weeks until urine output and solute excretion return to acceptable levels. If renal function does not return after 6 weeks of renal replacement therapy, recovery is unlikely and provisions should be made for long-term renal substitution therapy. Renal failure axioms are given in Table 5-3.

TABLE 5-3. Renal Failure Axioms

1. Clearances can be calculated using any timed urine sample; 24-hour collections are ideal but not necessary.
2. A diuretic trial is indicated if renal parenchymal disease is suspected. Use a large dose.
3. Renal failure is easy to detect but hard to admit.
4. Full nutrition is the systemic treatment for acute renal failure. Don't go without protein.
5. When planning renal replacement therapy, managing the extracellular fluid volume and solute toxicity are parallel but separate goals.

Pharmacology and ARF

Many drugs are excreted in whole or in part by the kidney. Serum levels of drugs that depend on renal excretion become elevated if renal function is compromised. If the drug has toxic side effects, this may have deleterious effects. Accordingly, drug dosages should be modified in patients in renal failure depending on the extent to which the drug is normally excreted by the kidney. A convenient nomogram for dealing with drug dosage in patients in renal failure is shown in Figure 5-7.

Monographs and Reviews

Bartlett RH, Bosch J, Geronemus R, Paganini E, Ronco C, Swartz R. Continuous arteriovenous hemofiltration for acute renal failure: workshop summary. Trans ASAIO 1988;34:67–77.
A summary of the methods for and the results of continuous hemofiltration presented at a 1988 American Society for Artificial Internal Organs (ASAIO) workshop.

Kramer P, ed. Arterio-venous hemofiltration. A kidney replacement therapy for the intensive care unit. Heidelberg, New York: Springer-Verlag, 1986.
Kramer invented the technique of continuous hemofiltration. This book contains a description of all the early studies and the technique.

5. Renal Physiology and Pathophysiology

LaGreca G, Fabris A, Ronco C, eds. CAVH, Proceedings of the International Symposium on Continuous Arteriovenous Hemofiltration. Milan: Wichtig Editore, 1986.
One of the early symposia on continuous renal replacement in the ICU.

Mault JR, Bartlett RH. Acute renal failure. In: Greenfield LJ, ed. Complications in surgery and trauma. Philadelphia: Lippincott, 1989:149–62.
This chapter describes the pathogenesis of ARF and the University of Michigan treatment algorithm.

Selected Reports

Abel RM, Beck CH, Abbot WM, et al. Improved survival from acute renal failure after treatment with intravenous essential L-amino acids and glucose: results of a prospective double-blind study. N Engl J Med 1973;208:695–9.
The first paper describing the infusion of essential amino acids (compared with no amino acids) in the treatment of ARF.

Bartlett RH, Mault JR, Dechert RE, Palmer J, Swartz RD, Port FK. Continuous arteriovenous hemofiltration: improved survival in surgical acute renal failure? Surgery 1986;100:400–8.
This study examined a large series of critically ill patients treated with continuous hemofiltration and full nutritional support and revealed survival was improved in those patients with ARF who had a positive caloric balance and were on a full feeding regimen.

Bywaters, EGL, Beall D. Crush injuries with impairment of renal function. Br Med J 1941;1:427–34.
The original description of ARF arising after nonrenal injury.

Cioffi WG, Taka A, Gamelli RL. Probability of surviving postoperative acute renal failure. Ann Surg 1984;200:205–11.

Corwin HL, Teplick RS, Schreiber MJ, et al. Prediction of outcome in acute renal failure. Am J Nephrol 1977;7:8–12.
These papers examine the survival rate in a typical series of patients with ARF.

Geronemous R, Schneider N. Continuous arteriovenous hemodialysis: a new modality for treatment of acute renal failure. Trans Am Soc Artif Intern Organs 1984;30:610–3.
This is the first description of the use of continuous hemofiltration in combination with simultaneous dialysis. This is the technique now used most widely in intensive care.

Kolff WJ, Berk HTJ. Artificial kidney: dialyzer with great area. Acta Med Scand 1994;117:121–34.
This classic paper is the first description of hemodialysis as a treatment for renal failure.

Martin PV, Dixon SM, Baker JD, et al. Risk of renal failure after major angiography. Arch Surg 1983;118:1417–20.
This paper reports the incidence and describes the possible causes of ARF after the injection of contrast medium.

Mault JR, Bartlett RH, Dechert RE, Clark SF, Swartz RD. Starvation: a major contributor to mortality in acute renal failure? Trans Am Soc Artif Intern Organs 1983; 29:390–4.

One of the first reports in which it was suggested that the mortality associated with ARF is related in part to withholding protein and caloric support.

Mault JR, Dechert RE, Lees P, Swartz RD, Port FK, Bartlett RH. Continuous arteriovenous filtration: an effective treatment for surgical acute renal failure. Surgery 1987;101:478–84.

A description of the technique of continuous arteriovenous hemofiltration in critically ill patients with ARF.

Mentzer SJ, Fryd DS, Kjellstrand CM. Why do patients with postsurgical acute tubular necrosis die? Arch Surg 1985;120:907–10.

This classic paper identifies isolated organ injury as the cause of the mortality associated with ARF. The study was done in renal transplant recipients who suffered ARF (as opposed to rejection). The mortality was 6%.

Sargent J, Gotch F, Borah M, et al. Urea kinetics: a guide to nutritional management of acute renal failure. Am J Clin Nutr 1978;31:1696–1702.

This classic paper describes the method for defining protein and urea kinetics in anuric and oliguric patients.

Teschan PE, Post RS, Smith LJ, et al. Post-traumatic renal insufficiency in military casualties. Am J Med 1955;18:172–86.

This classic paper is the first description of the use of hemodialysis for the treatment of posttraumatic ARF. This study was conducted near the frontlines during the Korean War.

6

Fluids and Electrolytes

The management of fluids and electrolytes is the simplest problem in all of critical care. It involves measuring or estimating the fluid and electrolyte losses on an 8- or 24-hour basis, then simply replacing what has been lost plus any prior deficits and any unusual anticipated extra losses. The normal requirements and losses are well known, and a standard set of commercially available fluids are available for infusion. The serum concentrations of electrolytes, proteins, and the components of various blood buffers are easily measured, although it is better to base management on the electrolyte losses than on their serum concentrations.

To manage fluids and electrolytes it is important to understand the anatomy and the kinetic physiology of body fluids and the small molecules that are dissolved therein. Without images of anatomy and physiology the entire fluid and electrolyte problem seems like a complex black box. Once the problem is visualized as anatomic spaces and daily balance diagrams, the black box falls away to reveal a few elementary components. The anatomy is diagrammed in Figure 6-1 and the kinetic physiology is diagrammed in Figure 6-4.

Body Composition

The total body water is divided in three anatomic spaces: the blood volume, the interstitial space, and the intracellular water. Within the blood volume, the plasma is part of the extracellular fluid and the red blood cell volume is part of the intracellular fluid, so that the system can be divided further into two compartments: intracellular water and extracellular water. The percentages of body weight shown in Figure 6-1 are accurate enough for the purpose of clinical calculation and are simple to remember. The extracellular water constitutes 20% of body weight and the intracellular water, 40% of body

156 Critical Care Physiology

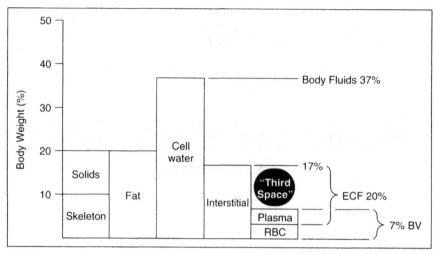

FIGURE 6-1. Body composition. (BV = blood volume; ECF = extracellular fluid.)

weight. The blood volume represents 7%, the interstitial space 17%, and the intracellular water 37% of body weight. (The skeleton [10%], fat-free solids [10%], and fat [20%] account for the remaining 40% of body weight.) It is useful to get in the habit of visualizing patients as if they were forced into this body composition diagram. A well-proportioned 80-kg man, for example, can be visualized as 50 kg of water divided into three compartments, surrounded by fat, and supported by the skeleton. Of the 50 liters of water, 33 liters are in cells. All of the metabolism under way in this patient is taking place within that 33 liters of water. The other 17 liters of water simply serve as the transport system to convey gases and nutrients back and forth from the outside environment to the cells. The 16 kg of skeleton and supporting tissues provides a framework for the metabolizing cells, and the 20 kg of fat is the reserve fuel for the metabolic processes. This mental image is fairly straightforward, but then consider a 40-year-old woman who is 5 feet (1.5 m) tall and weighs 300 pounds (135 kg). When considered in terms of the body composition diagram, there is a relatively small amount of total body water supporting a relatively small metabolizing cell mass, surrounded by a huge mound of fat. Or consider a 60-year-old man with cachexia stemming from carcinoma of the esophagus who is 6 feet (1.8 m) tall and weighs only 60 kg. His body fat represents only 5% of his body weight. The wasted muscle mass has resulted in a considerably decreased intracellular volume compared with his normal status. His total body water content and corresponding water compartments represent quite a large proportion of his body weight, but are actually much smaller than they were when he weighed 85 kg.

When visualizing a patient with the anatomic body composition shown in this diagram, it is useful to remember that the extracellular fluid is basically a sodium chloride solution and the intracellular fluid is basically a potassium phosphate solution. The cell membrane and the capillary membrane are identifiable in the diagram, and it is easy to envision the active and passive mechanisms that regulate the transport of water and other small molecules between the three spaces. For example, when 10 water molecules are injected into the plasma space, within minutes they will establish equilibrium between the three water compartments. Six molecules will be inside cells, three will be in the interstitial space, and one will remain in the plasma volume. The time it takes for equilibrium and the distribution of other molecules to occur depends on the size of the molecules and on the active and passive transport mechanisms. Ten sodium molecules will reach equilibrium in 30 minutes (depending to some extent on the plasma protein concentration), and one molecule might be inside a cell, six in the interstitial space, and three in the blood volume. Potassium, phosphate, and magnesium will mostly be in the intracellular fluid. Chloride, bicarbonate, and molecules larger than glucose or urea will be in the extracellular fluid.

Fluid and Electrolyte Losses

Once the anatomic spaces and the electrolyte composition of the spaces are visualized, it is easy to consider the interaction of the body fluid spaces with the external environment. Under normal conditions almost all interactions take place through the interstitial space (Figure 6-2). (The only exception is the loss of water vapor through the skin or the respiratory tract.) All normal body losses (urine, stool, tears, vomitus, and diarrhea) leave by way of the interstitial space, hence all these losses represent sodium chloride losses. Water, electrolytes, and nutrients are absorbed solely through the interstitial space in the intestine, with excess quantities excreted and an inadequate supply made up for by an endogenous metabolic rearrangement, all under endocrine control. Pathologic losses (bile, tissue fluid, pancreatic juice, pleural fluid, and blood) also take place through the interstitial space, hence all are variations of an isotonic sodium chloride solution. Pathologic losses, however, are generally replaced directly through the plasma volume in the form of intravenous fluids. One additional form of fluid electrolyte loss that must be considered is fluid temporarily lost to the extracellular compartments but still inside the patient. This is commonly referred to as *third-space loss* (meaning a third extracellular space, the first and second spaces being the plasma volume and interstitial fluids, respectively). Third-space loss occurs in the form of (1) localized edema after pancreatitis, thermal burn, or other inflammatory processes; (2) generalized edema after capillary leakage associated with sepsis or complement activation; or (3) the sequestration of fluid in body cavities such as the pleural space, peritoneum, or lumen of the

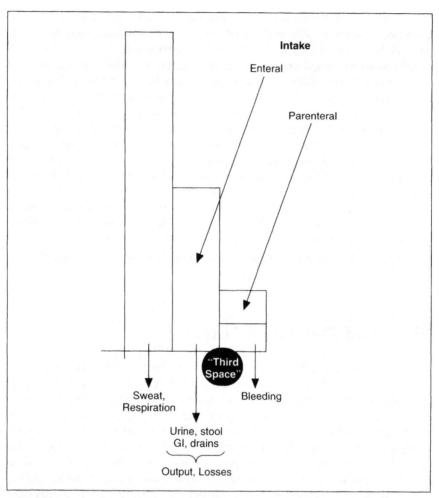

FIGURE 6-2. Fluid and electrolyte exchanges between the patient and the environment take place through the extracellular space, almost all through the interstitial component of the extracellular space.

gut. The electrolyte composition of third-space fluid is always that of plasma. The protein concentration is somewhere between that of plasma and interstitial fluid, usually closer to the latter. Third-space losses have to be replaced, just as do external losses, with the realization that the sequestered fluid and salt will eventually be resorbed and must be counted as output when it is lost and as intake when it is resorbed. Although extracellular losses are always sodium chloride based, the electrolyte idiosyncrasies of various fluids are an important component. The typical electrolyte compositions of various body fluids are shown in Table 6-1.

TABLE 6-1. Electrolyte Composition of Various Extracellular Space Fluids

Extracellular Fluids	Sodium (mEq/L)	Potassium (mEq/L)	Chloride (mEq/L)	Other (mEq/L)
Gastric fluid	20–120	15	130	H^+, 60
Bile	140	5	140	HCO_3^-, 44
Pancreatic fluid	140	5	70	HCO_3^-, 70
Ileostomy fluid	120	20	100	HCO_3^-, 40
Diarrhea	100	40	100	HCO_3^-, 40

Water and Electrolyte Balance

The kinetics of water and electrolytes are diagrammed in Figure 6-4. In a balance diagram, the intake that occurs over some specific period (typically 24 hours) is plotted from the baseline up (Figure 6-3). The output of that same fluid or electrolyte is plotted from the top of the intake line down. This brings the final result back to the baseline. The patient is in zero balance for that item over the 24-hour period. On a day with no intake, losses are plotted from the baseline down, with the resultant diagram showing a negative

FIGURE 6-3. In a balance diagram the intake is plotted from the baseline up and the output from that point back toward the baseline. In this example for water balance, the intake is 2 liters and the output, made up of urine, stool, and insensible losses, is 2 liters.

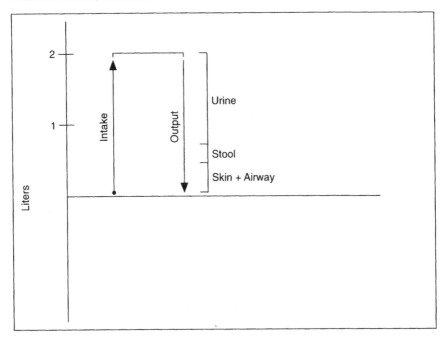

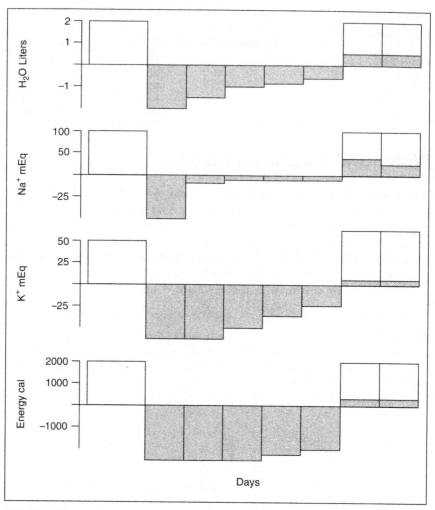

FIGURE 6-4. Balance diagram for water, sodium, and potassium and energy during a normal period, followed by a period of starving and thirsting. Positive or negative balance is shown in the shaded area.

balance. If there is more intake than loss, the balance will be shown to be positive. The balance diagram can be constructed for any substance, including water, electrolytes, protein (expressed as grams of nitrogen), or energy (expressed as calories). Figure 6-4 shows a balance diagram for water, sodium, potassium, energy, and nitrogen during a period of normal intake and output, starving and thirsting, a return to normal, and starving and thirsting plus stress or trauma.

In addition to the individual daily balance, the balance can be calculated as a cumulative balance over a longer time. The data from Figure 6-4 are plotted

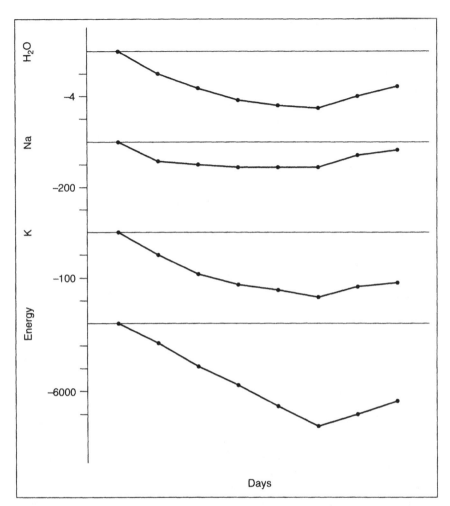

FIGURE 6-5. Cumulative balance diagram. The data from Figure 6-4 are replotted with a different scale.

as a cumulative balance in Figure 6-5. Calculations of both the cumulative and daily balances are very helpful in the management of patients. It is useful to construct a balance diagram, either on paper or mentally, for each day that a patient is in the intensive care unit. The electrolyte composition of external losses can be estimated or actually measured in the laboratory. The electrolyte composition of fluids given to the patient is known exactly. With this information the physician should keep the running balance diagram in mind daily. For example, it is useful to know that a given patient is in positive balance for 4 liters of water and 500 mEq of sodium and chloride over a 1-week period or that a patient is in a daily negative nitrogen balance despite some change in the nutritional regimen.

Fluid and Electrolyte Replacement

The fluids that are commonly used for intravenous infusion are listed in Table 6-2. Normal saline solution is designated "normal" because it is isotonic with human extracellular fluid. (It is not normal in the classic chemical sense of one gram equivalent per liter.) Normal saline solution consists of 9 g of sodium chloride in 1 liter of water. This 0.9% NaCl solution has 154 mEq/L each of sodium and chloride. Therefore it has an osmolarity of 308 mOsm/L (actually just slightly hypertonic). Although this solution is isotonic, it is certainly not normal in the sense of the electrolyte composition. However, it is very effective as an extracellular replacement, as long as it is borne in mind that an excess of chloride ions is given with each infusion.

A common solution that more closely resembles extracellular fluid is Hartman's solution, also known as *lactated Ringer's solution*. Ringer himself was a turn-of-the-century physiologist who devised this electrolyte solution by trial and error as a sustaining medium for the study of organs. By chance the final composition turned out to be quite close to that of human extracellular fluid, with the chloride excess problem solved by the substitution of sodium bicarbonate for 20% of the sodium chloride. Ringer's solution was used as an intravenous fluid, but it was not shelf stable because of the presence of bicarbonate ions. A New York pediatrician named Hartman had the wise idea of using sodium lactate instead of sodium bicarbonate to make up Ringer's solution. This solution is shelf stable for a long time, but the lactate molecules take up a hydrogen ion in the process of metabolism, so that it acts physiologically like bicarbonate. Thus lactated Ringer's or Hartman's solution (often referred to as the *balanced-salt solution*) is the mainstay of intravenous therapy when a large extracellular fluid loss must be replaced. It should be noted, however, that Dr. Hartman could have picked any small carbohydrate molecule that takes up a hydrogen ion during metabolism, such as acetate, citrate, or maleate. Presumably he picked sodium lactate because it was easily available to him. He never suspected that lactic acid accumulates during the metabolic acidosis resulting from ischemia or hypovolemia. This leads to the paradox of treating the lactic acidosis with infusions of lactated Ringer's solution, to the eternal confusion of medical students.

On many occasions it is necessary to give water without electrolytes intravenously to match hypotonic fluid losses. However, infusing water intravenously results in prompt and fatal hemolysis. This dilemma was solved (allegedly by Coller) using an isotonic solution of dextrose. This infusion can be given without the fear of hemolysis occurring, in that, as the dextrose is metabolized, "free" water is left to equilibrate in the total body water. A solution of 50 g of dextrose in 1 liter of water is isotonic. This is not called "normal dextrose," as one might expect, but rather 5% *dextrose in water*, commonly abbreviated as D5W. An alternative way of infusing a hypotonic

TABLE 6-2. Electrolyte Composition in One Liter of Common Parenteral Fluids

Intravenous	Sodium (mEq/L)	Potassium (mEq/L)	Chloride (mEq/L)	Glucose (g/L)	Protein (g/L)	Other
D5 0.9% NaCl	154	0	154	50	0	600 mOsm/L
D5 HNS; D5 0.45% NaCl	77	0	77	50	0	450 mOsm/L
Hartman (D5 lactated Ringer's solution)	130	4	109	50	—	Lactate 28 mEq/L, Ca 3 mEq/L
Standard TPN	35	40	53	250	4.25	Acetate 25 mEq/L, 1825 mOsm/L
Peripheral TPN	47	23	35	100	4.25	Acetate 36 mEq/L, 880 mOsm/L
0.1 Normal HCl	—	—	100	—	—	H^+, 100 mEq/L

HNS = half-normal saline; TPN = total parenteral nutrition.

electrolyte solution is to use one-half normal saline, which contains 4.5 g/L of sodium chloride, or 77 mEq/L of sodium and chloride each. This solution has an osmolarity of 152 mOsm/L, which is just at the borderline of hypotonicity that red blood cells can tolerate. Because of the risk of hemolysis, half-normal saline is always given as 5% dextrose in half-normal saline (D5 HNS). Obviously the osmolarity of D5 HNS is 452 mOsm/L, which is one and one-half times the normal osmolarity. Hypertonic fluids, however, do not cause hemolysis and are well tolerated. Fluids with an osmolarity greater than 800 mOsm/L are painful and irritating to peripheral veins and cause local thrombosis. For this reason, solutions with a tonicity exceeding 800 mOsm/L that require long-term infusion are administered into areas of rapidly flowing blood, particularly into the superior vena cava or right atrium. The observation that very hypertonic fluids can be administered safely into an area of rapid blood flow is attributed to Stanley Dudrick and his colleagues and forms the basis for all parenteral nutrition.

Patient Management

By comparing Tables 6-1 and 6-2 it is obvious that simply by keeping track of fluid and electrolyte losses and using well-characterized solutions for replacement, any desired daily balance for any of the various components can be achieved. Managing fluids and electrolytes then simply becomes an exercise in measuring output, estimating deficits and new losses, and matching intake to loss.

If losses of specific body fluids are excessive and not replaced, hypovolemia will eventuate, although all of the operative homeostatic mechanisms serve to maintain the blood volume at the expense of other body fluid compartments. The oncotic gradient created by proteins in the plasma space maintains salt and water in the vascular space whenever the capillary perfusion pressure dips below the oncotic pressure. Small amounts of hypovolemia trigger aldosterone and antidiuretic hormone production, thereby the water and sodium stores are conserved while potassium is selectively excreted. In this fashion a very long period of starvation, thirst, and catabolism is managed endogenously, with the hyperkaluria causing the potassium produced by cellular breakdown to be unloaded. During starvation, fat is metabolized, producing 1020 mL of water for each kilogram of fat metabolized, thus providing an endogenous source of water (albeit electrolyte-free water that will gradually dilute the electrolyte concentration of extracellular fluid). In addition to simple hypovolemia, extracellular fluid losses can lead to specific electrolyte deficiencies depending on the fluids lost. For example, bile contains 44 mEq/L of bicarbonate, so that an extensive bile loss may lead to systemic acidosis stemming from loss of bicarbonate buffer. This situation is exacerbated if the bile loss is replaced using sodium chloride solutions. Similarly, gastric juice typically contains more than 100 mEq/L of hydrogen ions and 15 to 20 mEq/L of potassium ions, all present as the chloride salt. Therefore prolonged vomiting leads to hypokalemic, hypochloremic metabolic alkalosis. This situation would be exacerbated if the gastric losses were replaced by D5W. The various combinations of high or low concentrations of sodium, potassium, chloride, and magnesium are discussed in great detail in standard textbooks. A single measurement of serum electrolytes can characterize the clinical picture, then management consisting simply of calculating intake and output and replacing the deficit proceeds easily. Although measuring the serum electrolyte levels is useful for identifying abnormal or deficit states, it is generally not useful or necessary for managing the fluids and electrolytes in a routine patient. If laboratory measurements are to be made, it is much more useful to measure the electrolyte composition in external losses (urine, wound drainage, diarrhea, and vomitus) than it is to try and guess what the actual losses were based on changes in the serum electrolyte levels.

The use of all this information to manage fluids and electrolytes on a typical patient is demonstrated in Figure 6-6. The first step is to calculate the water, sodium, potassium, chloride, calories, and protein requirements for the next 24 hours. In each of these categories the basic daily maintenance, the deficit replacement if any, the expected losses if any, and special nutritional requirements need to be determined. The second step is to sum the quantities in each category to determine the total requirements for 24 hours. In the third step the amount and type of replacement fluid necessary to achieve these requirements have to be determined for each of the categories of fluids and electrolytes. The oral intake, amount provided by parenteral nutrition, and specific replacement must be included, and the total water requirement is completed with D5 HNS. Step four consists of totaling the quantities in each category to determine the total intake for 24 hours. Of course the rate and type of fluid infusion may have to be adjusted as the day progresses, depending on actual losses. A simple method for uncomplicated fluid and electrolyte replacement is to use D5 HNS plus 20 mEq/L of potassium chloride given at a rate of 1 mL/kg/hr. This supplies 24 mL of water per kilogram of body weight per day and 1.8 mEq of sodium, 0.5 mEq potassium, and 4.8 cal per kilogram per day. Typical basic maintenance of the water volume is shown in Figure 6-7.

Acid-Base Physiology

Acid-base relationships as related to the bicarbonate buffer system are depicted in Figure 6-8. Because the bicarbonate buffer is the dominant buffer in body fluids, acid-base relationships are always shown in this context. Henderson and Hasselbalch derived an equation based on the pH of the bicarbonate buffer, which basically states that the pH of a bicarbonate buffer solution will be 7.44 when the ratio of bicarbonate ions to carbonic acid ions

Fluid and Electrolyte Management Algorithm
(75 Kg Estimated Dry Weight) Typical Example

1. Calculate requirements for 24 hours

	H₂O	Sodium (Na)	Potassium (K)	Chloride (Cl)	Calories	Protein	Example
Basic daily maintenance	2250	75	37	60	1875	75	Urine and insensible
Deficit replacement	1000	140	10	100	-	-	GI loss
Expected losses	1000	140	5	100	-	-	Third space
Nutrition					?	?	

2. Total requirements

3. Calculate replacement fluids

	H₂O	Sodium (Na)	Potassium (K)	Chloride (Cl)	Calories	Protein	Other
Oral, enteral, and parenteral nutrition	1000	35	18	53	1000	4.25	(Standard TPN)
Specific replacement	1000	130	4	109	200	0	D5LR
Balance D5 ½ NS	1000	77	0	77	200	0	D5HNS

4. Total infusion

Simple starter:
D5 ½ NS + 20KCl @ 1 cc/Kg/hr = 24 cc/Kg H₂O/day
1.8 mEq Na/Kg/d
.5 mEq K/Kg/d
4.8 cal/Kg/d

FIGURE 6-6. To calculate the type and dosage of intravenous fluids, categorize and sum the requirements, then the amount of replacement solutions needed. (D5 1/2NS = 5% dextrose in half-normal saline solution; D5LR = lactated Ringer's solution.)

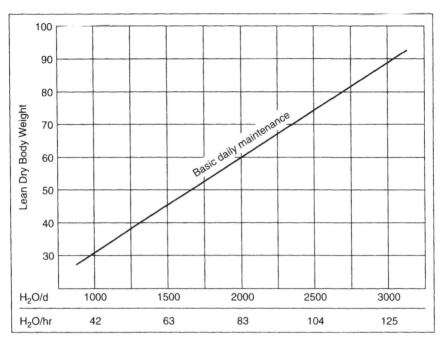

FIGURE 6-7. Maintenance water requirements based on lean body weight.

is 20 to 1. All of the various diagrams and nomograms describing acid-base physiology are essentially variations on the Henderson-Hasselbalch equation. Five of these variations are shown in Figures 6-8 to 6-12. The equation shown in Figure 6-8 is currently the most valuable version because the pH and partial pressure of CO_2 ($P{CO_2}$) variables are always reported as part of modern blood gas measurement (the bicarbonate measurement with this system is calculated rather than measured). Because the $P{CO_2}$ represents the carbonic acid concentration, fluctuations in pH at various levels of $P{CO_2}$ represent either respiratory alkalosis or acidosis, whereas fluctuations in pH at a constant $P{CO_2}$ represent metabolic alterations.

There are two archaic terms that have persisted into the modern era without much justification: *base deficit* and *anion gap*. *Base deficit* is a way of describing the difference between the measured serum bicarbonate level and the normal value of 27 mEq/L, which actually represents the ionic equivalent of all the CO_2 in blood, including the bicarbonate and carbonic acid. This measurement system was used by Siggaard-Anderssen in the 1960s when he was particularly interested in metabolic alkalosis (see Figure 6-12). The patients he was studying had a serum bicarbonate level in the 30 to 40-mEq/L range, so he expressed the abnormality as a 3- to 13-mEq/L "base excess." The concept of describing the difference between the measured bicarbonate level and the normal value is a very useful bedside shorthand method to characterize acid-base disorders, so this term has persisted.

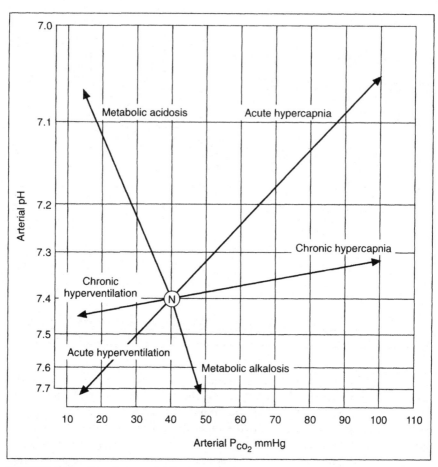

FIGURE 6-8. Bicarbonate buffer system plotted as the pH and P_{CO_2}.

However, research interest subsequently shifted from alkalotic to acidotic states, particularly the metabolic acidosis caused by inadequate tissue perfusion and anaerobic metabolism, with the accumulation of hydrogen ions and lactate, as discussed earlier. To describe the condition of metabolic acidosis, researchers borrowed Siggaard-Anderssen's convenient terminology, which unfortunately translated into the term *negative base excess* when referring to acidosis. This terminology has persisted into the modern era, although it would be much better to describe such abnormalities as a "buffer base deviation," as several authors have proposed.

If one adds together the easily measurable cations (sodium and potassium) and the easily measurable anions (chloride and bicarbonate), then subtracts the anion measurement from the cation measurement, the difference is approximately 10 mEq/L. This difference is correctly assumed to represent the anionic charges on protein molecules (give or take a few of the

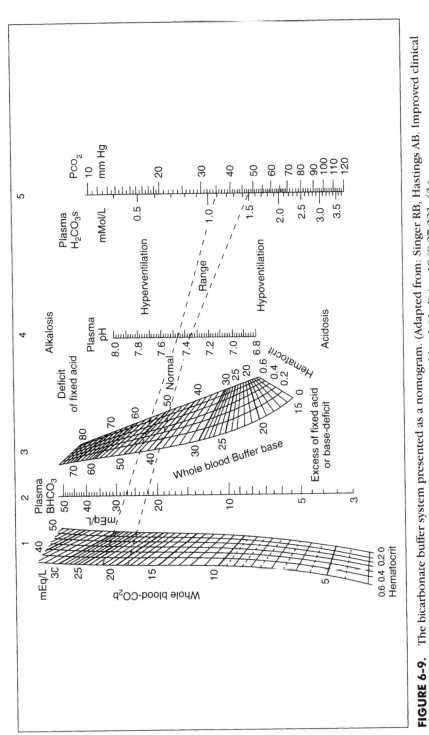

FIGURE 6-9. The bicarbonate buffer system presented as a nomogram. (Adapted from: Singer RB, Hastings AB. Improved clinical method for estimation of disturbances of acid-base balance in human blood. Medicine 1948;27:223–42.)

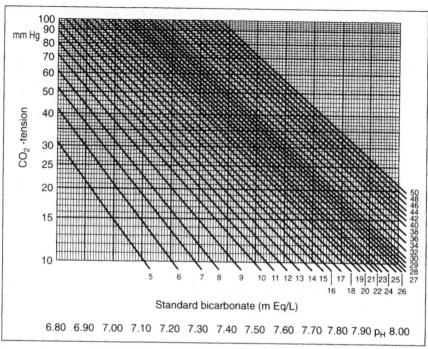

FIGURE 6-10. The bicarbonate buffer system in a plot showing relationship of P_{CO_2}, bicarbonate, and pH in plasma of normal protein content but varying base content. (From: Astrup P. Scand J Clin Lab Invest 1956;8:33.)

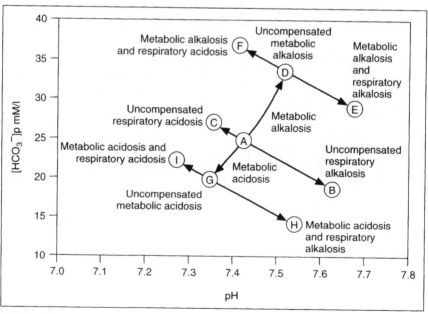

FIGURE 6-11. The bicarbonate buffer system plotted as bicarbonate and pH. A = normal. (From Davenport HW, ed. The ABC of acid-base chemistry, 4th ed. Chicago: The University of Chicago Press, 1958.)

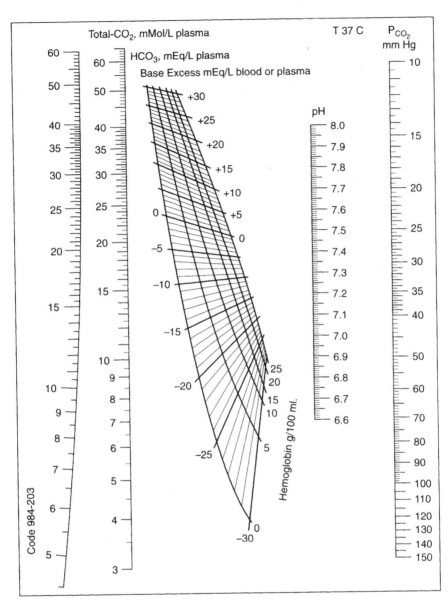

FIGURE 6-12. The bicarbonate buffer system presented as a nomogram by Siggaard-Anderssen. The "base excess" is introduced in the Siggaard-Anderssen nomogram. (From: Siggaard-Anderssen O. The acid base status of the blood, 4th ed. Copenhagen: Munksgaard, 1963.)

lesser salts and minerals). If an acid accumulates in the blood, the hydrogen ion is not accounted for on the cation side but the decrease in bicarbonate buffer compensation would appear as a bicarbonate deficit on the anion side. Suppose that a patient had 10 mEq/L of hydrogen ions because of lactic acidosis with ischemia, or an excess of sulfuric and phosphoric acid because of renal failure, or a toxic level of acetylsalicylic acid because of overdose, the calculated "anion gap" would then be 20 mEq/L. Thus metabolic acidosis can be described in terms of an "increased anion gap," which is simply another way of saying that the serum bicarbonate level is less than 27 mEq/L.

The treatment of acid-base imbalance is always correctly said to consist of treating the underlying cause of the problem. Replacing deficits, compensating for continuing losses, and resuscitating from hypovolemia constitute the appropriate first-line treatment for obstructing duodenal ulcer, intractable diarrhea, hemorrhagic shock, and so on. These maneuvers will, in time, correct any acid-base imbalance, assuming that the patient's kidney function is normal and the basic anatomic or physiologic problem is corrected. However, there are situations in which it is not safe to wait for endogenous compensation to occur but instead to treat the acid-base abnormalities directly. The treatment of respiratory acidosis or alkalosis is simply a matter of adjusting the alveolar ventilation. The treatment of metabolic acidosis is accomplished by the infusion of bicarbonate or other buffers, and the treatment of metabolic alkalosis is accomplished by the infusion of acid.

The treatment of metabolic acidosis, at one time thought to be essential to ensure normal cellular functioning, is now controversial. It is clear that acidosis per se is not detrimental to otherwise normal people, even to the extreme. We have all seen patients with a pH of 6.8 to 7.0 lasting for 12 hours or more who are in a state of severe respiratory acidosis but who recover promptly and without organ dysfunction as soon as their P_{CO_2} is normalized. On the other hand, a patient with a metabolic acidosis below 7.0 for an hour or two will suffer multiple-organ failure and usually die. The cause of organ failure and death in this patient is obviously not the acidosis but the ischemia or hypovolemia that led to it. Nonetheless, resuscitation from profound hypovolemia seems to proceed more quickly and the response to inotropic and vasopressor drugs seems greater when pH is normalized. For this reason it is common practice to give sodium bicarbonate solution as a temporizing treatment in patients with severe metabolic acidosis. (For reasons of shelf stability, sodium lactate or sodium acetate can be used, although the carbohydrate molecule must be metabolized before any buffering effect is realized.) To determine the amount of bicarbonate required to treat acidosis, assume that the bicarbonate is distributed in the extracellular space only. This will obviously be an underestimate of the amount of buffer required, as the hydrogen ion is distributed throughout the total body water. The amount of bicarbonate that will bring the bicarbonate concentration back to 27 mEq/L can be calculated roughly as the buffer base deviation times 25% of the body weight. If this amount of buffer is given as sodium bicarbonate, a very

TABLE 6-3. Fluid and Electrolyte Axioms

1. Normal extracellular fluid losses are replenished with half-normal saline. Excess sodium causes edema.
2. Replace crystalloid with crystalloid, plasma with plasma, blood with blood. Corollary: the saline replacement of blood and plasma loss requires 3 : 1 replacement and causes anasarca.
3. Four organs malfunction when edematous: lung, brain, gut, and heart.
4. Abnormal losses are variations of extracellular fluid and hence can be replaced with saline solutions.
5. For accurate management, measure the electrolyte levels in fluid losses not in serum.
6. When saline solutions are used to replace third-space losses, the third space will be as large as the amount of fluid given.
7. Do not confuse the extracellular space with the blood volume. Corollary: the pulmonary capillary wedge pressure is not a measure of fluid overload or underload.

heavy sodium load will be infused. If a sodium overload already exists or if the patient is in renal failure, an alternative is to use TRIS (tromethamine, THAM). THAM is prepared at a concentration of 36 g/L and has buffering properties of approximately 1 mEq/mL in this concentration.

Metabolic alkalosis requires treatment only if the pH exceeds 7.7 (to treat tetany or seizures) or if the patient is being weaned from a mechanical ventilator and has a pronounced metabolic alkalosis. The amount of hydrochloric acid required for infusion is determined in the same fashion as the dose of bicarbonate for the treatment of acidosis, that is, the buffer base deviation in milliequivalents per liter times 25% of the body weight. Hydrochloric acid is usually given as 0.1 normal HCl, which has 100 mEq/L hydrogen ions and chloride ions per liter (Table 6-3).

Monographs and Reviews

Cannon WB. Organization for physiological homeostasis. Physiol Rev 1929;9:399–431.
This landmark publication introduces the term homeostasis *and includes all the appropriate references to Pfluger, Bernard, Haldane, Henderson, Gamble, and others who developed the concept.*

Davenport HW, ed. The ABC of acid-base chemistry, 4th ed. Chicago: The University of Chicago Press, 1958.
This classic monograph made acid-base physiology understandable to every generation of medical students and physicians since it was first published in 1947. Even today it remains mandatory reading in any critical care curriculum.

Fabri PJ. Fluids and electrolyte physiology and pathophysiology. In: Miller TA, ed. Physiologic basis of modern surgical care. St. Louis: Mosby, 1989.
A recent review of fluid physiology.

Gamble JL. Chemical anatomy, physiology, and pathology of extracellular fluid. Boston: Department of Pediatrics, Harvard Medical School, 1942.
The classic original description of body fluid spaces and their composition described in "Gamblegrams."

Moore FD. Metabolic care of the surgical patient. Philadelphia: Saunders, 1956.
The classic reference on normal and abnormal body spaces, fluids, and electrolytes. Although the text refers to surgical patients, the discussion is applicable to all critically ill patients.

Moore FD, Olesen KH, McMurray JD, et al. The body cell mass and its supporting environment. Philadelphia: Saunders, 1963.
This is the summary of all the work on the isotopic dilution of body fluid spaces conducted by Francis Moore's research group and is the classic reference on the methods and the results.

Selected Reports

Astrup P, Jorgensen K, Siggaard-Anderssen O, et al. The acid-base metabolism: a new approach. Lancet 1960;1:1035–40.
Description of the pH log P_{CO_2} graph.

Brimioulle S, Berre J, Dufaye P, et al. Hydrochloric acid infusion for treatment of metabolic alkalosis associated with respiratory acidosis. Crit Care Med 1989;17:232–6.
Treatment of metabolic alkalosis is only necessary when a pH of greater than 7.7 leads to tetany or when weaning a patient from a ventilator. This paper describes the authors' experience with hydrochloric acid infusion to buffer metabolic alkalosis

Coller FA, Campbell KN, Vaughan HH, et al. Postoperative salt intolerance. Ann Surg 1944;119:533–42.
The use of 5% dextrose is proposed as a way to give water without sodium to postoperative patients.

Demling RH, Manohar M, Will JA, et al. The effect of plasma oncotic pressure on the pulmonary micro-circulation after hemorrhagic shock. Surgery 1979;86:323–31.
In experiments on sheep, the oncotic gradient between plasma and interstitial fluid was found to be maintained during progressive hemodilution until the albumin level was less than 1.5 g/dL.

Henderson LJ. The theory of neutrality regulation in the animal organism. Am J Physiol 1903;21:427–35.
The description of the bicarbonate buffer system on which the Henderson-Hasselbalch equation is based.

Huckabee WE. Abnormal resting lactate: I. Significance in hospital patients. Am J Med 1961;30:838–45.
The classic original description of lactate as the acid accumulating in the setting of metabolic acidosis.

Lyons LJ, Owns JH, Moore FD. Posttraumatic alkalosis: incidence and pathophysiology of alkalosis in surgery. Surgery 1966;60:93–101.
A report describing the incidence of the most common abnormality of acid-base balance in the intensive care unit; in it the term buffer-base deviation *is introduced.*

Moore FD. Determination of total body water and solids with isotopes. Science 1946;104:157–60.

The original description of isotope dilution techniques in humans; it served as the basis for body composition research and the beginning of nuclear medicine.

Powers SR, Shah D, Ryond D, et al. Hypertonic mannitol in the therapy of acute respiratory distress syndrome. Ann Surg 1977;185:619–26.

One of the first papers demonstrating improvement in pulmonary function with forced diuresis in the treatment of the adult respiratory distress syndrome.

Siggaard-Anderssen O. The acid base status of the blood, 4th ed. Copenhagen: Munksgaard, 1963.

The Siggaard-Anderssen nomogram describes a deviation from normal pH as a base excess.

Singer RB, Hastings AB. Improved clinical method for estimation of disturbances of acid-base balance in human blood. Medicine 1948;27:223–42.

One of the nomograms describing the bicarbonate buffer system.

Virgilio RW, Rice CL, Smith DE, et al. Crystalloid vs colloid resuscitation: is one better? Surgery 1979;85:129.

A very well controlled clinical study of colloid versus crystalloid replacement for the treatment of blood loss during aortic operations. Patients were resuscitated to a standardized wedge pressure. The crystalloid replacement required was three times that of colloid replacement, but colloid resuscitation required fine tuning to prevent congestive heart failure.

Wangensteen OW, Paine JR. Treatment of acute intestinal obstruction by suction with a duodenal tube. JAMA 1933;101:153–8.

Wangensteen's classic paper on intestinal decompression and intravenous fluid management in the setting of intestinal obstruction.

7

Nervous System

Viewed in its simplest terms, the entire purpose of intensive care is to keep the brain alive and healthy during the impairment or failure of other organ systems. Treatment of the nervous system is aimed almost entirely at maintaining adequate function of the other vital organs. Aside from treating central nervous system infection and preventing brain ischemia and high intracranial pressure, the attention given to the nervous system primarily consists of monitoring to be sure it is still functioning well and ensuring adequate function of the other organ systems.

The nature of brain and spinal cord disorders and the management of peripheral neuropathy in critically ill patients are beyond the scope of this handbook, and the physiologic and pathophysiologic characteristics of brain function and malfunction are not discussed in any detail here. The figures in the handbook and supplementary discussion in this chapter are intended to provide a readily accessible reference to neurologic localization and a beginning approach to the management of cerebral perfusion, seizures, coma, and traumatic head injury.

Level of Consciousness

The Glasgow coma scale has become the standard way of characterizing the level of consciousness. Calculating the score involves the simple evaluation of the patient's best motor function, best verbal response, and best eye response. A normal alert, awake person who can respond to commands with eyes open at rest gets an arbitrary score of 6 for the motor response, 5 for the verbal response, and 4 for the eye response, for a total score of 15. A flaccid, comatose person whose eyes are closed and who shows no response to verbal commands and no motor function gets a score of 1 in each category, for a total score of 3. Various neurologic findings according to a score of from 1 to the highest score in each grading category are listed in Table 7-1. This score is converted to commonly observed clinical situations in Table 7-2. In general a patient with a Glasgow coma score of 9 or greater responds to stimuli and appears close to full consciousness. A patient with a Glasgow coma score of 8 or less is comatose and unresponsive and shows variable responses to pain. Verbal responses scoring 3 to 5 and motor responses scoring 5 or 6 require that the patient be able to speak. Obviously a patient who is intubated or has a tracheostomy cannot speak, so the score assigned is based on the observer's best estimate of how the patient could respond verbally if he or she were able to or the patient is given the lower score with a "T" added to indicate that full evaluation was not possible.

TABLE 7-1. Physical Examination Findings as Correlated with Brain Level and Glasgow Coma Score

Level of Consciousness	Brain Level	Glasgow Scale			Defect	
		Motor	Verbal	Eye	Metabolic	Anatomic
Alert, responds, opens eyes	All normal	6	5	4	—	—
Confused, disoriented	Cortex	5	4		—	—
Inappropriate words	Cortex		3		—	—
Eyes open to sound	Cortex			3	—	—
Withdraws to pain	Cortex	4			—	—
Makes sounds, no words	Cortex		2		—	—
Eyes open to pain	Cortex			2	—	—
Eyes closed, no response to sound	Midbrain		1	1	—	—
Decorticate (flexor) posture	Midbrain	3			—	—
Pupillary reflex	Midbrain				Present	Absent
Decerebrate (extensor) posture	Pons	2			—	—
Doll's eyes reflex	Pons				Present	Absent
Cold nystagmus reflex	Pons				Present	Absent
Flaccid to pain	Medulla	1			—	—
Spontaneous respiration only	Medulla				—	—

TABLE 7-2. Typical Glasgow Score Range

Alert, awake, oriented, eyes open	15
Confused, speaks, opens eyes to sound	12
Unconscious but responds to stimulus (moves, opens eyes, makes sound)	10
Unconscious, withdraws or grimaces in response to pain	6
Unconscious, flexes in response to pain only	5
Flaccid	3

TABLE 7-3. Common Causes of Coma

Medications: sedatives, analgesics, anesthetics	Mechanical
Metabolic and toxic	Trauma, raised intracranial pressure
Hypoglycemia, hyperglycemia	Venous thrombosis, occlusion
Hyponatremia, hypernatremia	Arterial embolus, thrombus, bleeding
Uremia	Hydrocephalus
Liver failure	Subdural, epidural hematoma
Alcohol, other drugs	Meningioma and benign tumors
Anoxia, hypercapnia	Malignancy
Microbiologic	Primary brain tumors
Meningitis	Metastatic tumors
Encephalitis	

Evaluation of the causes of coma in patients with a Glasgow coma score of 8 or less is illustrated in Tables 7-1 and 7-3. The first step in evaluating the comatose patient is to distinguish coma resulting from anatomic brain injury from coma resulting from drugs, uremia, liver failure, or other metabolic causes. This is initially differentiated on the basis of the pupillary reflexes, doll's eyes reflex, and nystagmus in response to cold stimulation of the middle ear. If all three of these pons- and brainstem–mediated reflexes are intact, then coma is most likely of metabolic origin. If all of these reflexes are absent, major brain injury at the level of the upper brainstem is present. If the eye and nystagmus reflexes are equivocal or indeterminate, the cause of the coma may be a combination of metabolic causes and anatomic injury such as the hypoxic-ischemic injury that occurs after cardiac arrest or profound hypoxia. In addition, findings may be equivocal in patients in a coma secondary to trauma, intracranial bleeding, or infection such as meningitis or viral encephalitis. In this circumstance, lumbar puncture or fluid sampling, electroencephalography, computed tomographic (CT) scanning, and magnetic resonance imaging are required to determine the cause of coma. Some of the common causes of coma are categorized and summarized in Table 7-3.

Spinal Cord Levels

Critically ill patients may have a spinal cord or peripheral nerve injury that is either known to exist or is suspected, making understanding of the sensory dermatomes and motor innervation at different levels of the cord important for the intensive care physician. These cord levels with their appropriate sensory and motor correlates are outlined in Table 7-4.

Cerebral Blood Flow

Blood flow to the brain is remarkably well autoregulated over a wide range of blood perfusion pressures. The relationship between perfusion and cerebral

TABLE 7-4. Sensory and Motor Levels in the Spinal Cord

Cord levels	Sensory	Nerves	Motor
C4	Shoulder	—	—
C5	Outer arm	Musculocutaneous	Biceps
C6	Thumb	Radial	Extensors
C7	Middle finger	Median	Flexors
C8	Little finger	Ulnar	Interossei
T1	Inner arm	—	—
T4	Nipple	—	—
T10	Umbilicus	—	—
T11	Gonads	—	—
L1	Hip	—	—
L2	Thigh	Obturator	Adductors
L3	Knee	Femoral	Quadriceps
L4	Inner calf	Tibial	Gastrocnemius
L5	Big toe	Peroneal	Toe extensors
S1	Little toe	—	—
S4	Anal	—	Anal sphincter

blood flow under normal conditions and during hyperventilation and hypoventilation is shown in Figure 7-1. The cerebral perfusion pressure is the mean arterial pressure minus the intracranial pressure. Obviously it is necessary to measure the intracranial pressure to calculate the cerebral perfusion pressure. This is done by inserting a catheter or a pressure-sensitive device through the skull into the epidural space, subdural space, brain parenchyma, or lateral ventricle. The normal intracranial pressure varies with respiration; therefore it is properly measured at the functional residual capacity. Usually the respiratory effect is minimal and the intracranial pressure is expressed as the mean intracranial pressure by damping down the respiratory variation. The normal intracranial pressure is less than 10 mm Hg (13.6 cm H_2O). The normal mean arterial pressure is 80 mm Hg, so that normal cerebral perfusion pressure is approximately 70 mm Hg. Under these conditions, cerebral blood flow is normal (50 mL/100 g of brain tissue/min). Autoregulation maintains this level of normal cerebral blood flow despite wide swings in arterial blood pressure and during moderate elevations of intracranial pressure. This is shown in Figure 7-1. However, if the arterial pressure is low and the cerebral pressure is high, some regions of the brain may experience decreased cerebral blood flow, which can result in ischemia or infarction. In conditions in which elevated intracranial pressure is suspected (for example, head trauma, subarachnoid hemorrhage, encephalitis, meningitis, and Reye's syndrome), it is worth the small risk of infection to place an intracranial pressure monitor to assess the intracranial pressure, thus allowing calculation of the cerebral perfusion pressure. An elevated intracranial pressure is treated by osmotic agents such as urea or mannitol that do not cross the normal blood-brain barriers and by elevating the head, thereby minimizing the intrathoracic pressure.

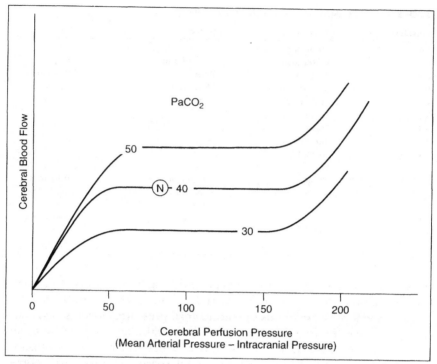

FIGURE 7-1. Autoregulation maintains cerebral blood flow constant over a wide range of cerebral perfusion pressures. CO_2 acts as a vasodilator on the resistance arterioles of the brain.

TABLE 7-5. An Algorithm for Treatment of Acute Seizures in the Intensive Care Unit Patient

Metabolic causes: hypoglycemia, hypoxia
Diazepam (Valium), 10–40 mg intravenously
Phenobarbital, 1 mg/kg intravenously up to 10 mg/kg total
Phenytoin (Dilantin), 500 mg intravenously up to 15 mg/kg total

Seizures

When seizures occur in patients in the intensive care unit, the cause is most commonly related to hypoxia, hypoglycemia, or electrolyte imbalance, specifically hyponatremia. In metabolic disorders, continuous or irregular muscle twitching and fasciculation can resemble seizures, and sometimes electroencephalography is required to differentiate neuromuscular excitation from brain-induced seizures. Benzodiazapenes such as Valium (diazepam) or Ativan (lorazepam) are usually effective in stopping seizures acutely. Dilantin and barbiturates are used for both acute and chronic control. An

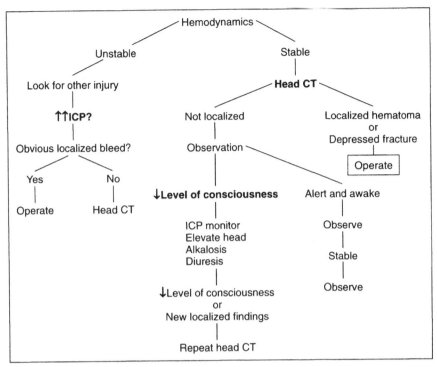

FIGURE 7-2. An algorithm for the evaluation and management of head trauma. (ICP = intracranial pressure.)

algorithm for the treatment of acute seizures in intensive care unit patients is shown in Table 7-5.

Head trauma is a common problem in patients in surgical intensive care units. A sudden deterioration in brain function after trauma may be caused by a hematoma, which demands urgent surgical drainage. However the CT scan has replaced exploratory drill holes and runs to the operation room as the diagnostic tool. Any hospital that treats trauma patients should be organized to do emergency head CT scanning within minutes in emergency room or intensive care unit patients. An algorithm for the treatment of head injury is shown in Figure 7-2.

Monographs and Reviews

Arbit E, Krol G. Coma, seizures and brain death. In: Wilmore DW, Brennan MF, Harken AF, Holcroft JW, Meakins JL, eds. Care of the surgical patient. New York: Scientific American Medicine, 1994.
A recent concise review of the brain problems encountered in the critically ill patient.

Marion DW. The Glasgow coma scale score: contemporary application. Intensive Care World 1994;11:101–2.
A brief update on the use of the Glasgow coma score in intensive care.

McGillicuddy JE. Cerebral protection: pathophysiology and treatment of increased intracranial pressure. Chest 1985;87:85–93.
An excellent review of intracranial pressure monitoring and management techniques.

Watling SM, Dasta JF. Prolonged paralysis in intensive care unit patients after the use of neuromuscular blocking agents: a review of the literature. Crit Care Med 1994;22:884–93.
An excellent review of the literature on prolonged neuromuscular blockade with and without steroids, together with recommendations for monitoring and prevention.

Selected Reports

Benzer A, Mitterschiffthaler G, Maros M, et al. Prediction of non-survival after trauma. Innsbruck coma scale. Lancet 1991;388:977–82.

Levy DE, Bates D, Carrona JJ. Prognosis in non-traumatic coma. Ann Intern Med 1981;94:293–310.
These two papers describe the likelihood of recovery after severe brain injury.

Firsching SR, Friedman WA. Multimodality evoked potentials and early prognosis in comatose patients. Neurosurg Rev 1990;13:141–9.
Description of evoked potentials as a way to evaluate injury and prognosis in a patient in a coma.

Griffin D, Fairman N, Coursin D, et al. Acute myopathy during treatment of status asthmaticus with corticosteroids and steroidal muscle relaxant. Chest 1992;102:510–4.
A report of three cases and literature review of 15 similar cases implicating the steroidal muscle relaxants (pancuronium and vecuronium) as a cause of acute myopathy.

Kaufman HH, Bretaudiere JP, Rowlands BJ, et al. General metabolism in head injury. J Neurosurg 1987;20:254–65.
An excellent study of the caloric and protein energy requirements and of metabolism in 76 patients with head injury.

Teasdale G, Jennett B. Assessment of coma and impaired consciousness. Lancet 1974;2:81–8.
The original description of the Glasgow coma scoring system.

8

Host Defenses

Injury and infection are problems for every critically ill patient, either as the cause of the illness or as a potential complication. Normal physiologic systems that stop bleeding, prevent infection, and heal tissues are constantly at work in the critically ill patient. Malfunction of these systems is manifested as bleeding, infection, too much or too little inflammation, and too much or too little fibrosis. The three host defense systems *thrombosis, inflammation, and healing* are interdependent and balance themselves through a remarkable network of intercellular chemical mediators that act locally but may produce systemic symptoms. The timing of events after tissue injury is a fascinating phenomenon. The activation and response of platelets occurs in seconds, fibrin formation in minutes, inflammation in hours, fibrinolysis (and infection, if it occurs) in days, and fibrosis and healing in weeks. This complex system may be activated by direct tissue injury, sterile inflammation (as in pancreatitis, thermal burns, or shock), bacteria- or virus-induced inflammation, or chronic inflammation and fibrosis without apparent cause (rheumatoid arthritis). In critically ill patients we have a good understanding of the appropriate management to implement for the control of bleeding problems. We can culture the full spectrum of infectious microorganisms, and we have drugs to kill most of them (the drugs are so effective that we sometimes forget about drainage and debridement as treatments). We are just beginning to understand the chemical phenomena underlying the systemic response to inflammation. Although many drugs for inhibiting these mediators are on the horizon, the only potent inflammatory inhibitor currently available (corticosteroids) does more harm than good in most critically ill patients. We pay little attention to the tissue-healing phase of host defense. This is probably because we have no effective way of enhancing healing when it is defective and no safe way to inhibit healing when it is excessive.

To serve as an example of host defenses in the critically ill patient, let us consider the case of a young man who has been stabbed in the right flank. The knife wound has gone through the skin, abdominal wall, right colon, and inferior vena cava. Through a separate midline incision the vena cava has been repaired, stool washed out from the abdomen, and a double-barreled diverting colostomy done. The patient has received five units of packed red blood cells and 7 liters of salt solution. He has received one prophylactic dose of cephalosporin and aminoglycoside, and he is now being admitted to the intensive care unit (ICU) with stable vital signs.

Bleeding and Clotting

As soon as the knife cut through blood vessels the *activation of platelets* began, stimulated by two mechanisms: (1) shear stress caused by a disruption in the normal laminar flow of blood and (2) contact with collagen in the vessel walls and tissues. Shear stress causes a conformational change in the phospholipid surface of the platelet, exposing adherent molecules called *receptors*. Collagen causes a similar conformational change, exposing adherent molecules called *1A receptors*. These receptors stick to the collagen in the cut and raw surfaces outside the endothelium, resulting in platelet adhesion. An intermediary protein molecule known as the *von Willebrand factor* facilitates this adhesion. When the platelet has adhered, materials from the granules in the platelets are expelled through the platelet membrane. These granules contain many compounds, including thromboxane, serotonin and bradykinin (all of which cause local vessel constriction), as well as platelet factor 4, which stimulates the adhesion of other platelets. Like tissue thromboplastic factor, platelet factor 4 initiates the conversion of Factor X to Xa in the fibrin formation sequence. Each successive platelet undergoes a similar adhesion and activation reaction, and a sizable platelet aggregate forms all around the cut surfaces.

In the plasma surrounding the platelets in the aggregate, a sequential series of enzymatic reactions takes place, leading in a minute or so to the *formation of fibrin*, a gluey, ropey polymer that attaches to and stabilizes the platelet aggregate as it grows (by activation of the platelet receptor 2B3A). The enzymes in this sequence are identified by roman numerals and also by specific names either describing their function or referring to their discoverer. Any one of the enzymes can be deficient or inhibited, leading to the delay or inhibition of fibrin formation. As already noted, the fibrin formation sequence is initiated by the platelet thromboplastic factor or the tissue thromboplastic factor, or both. Both factors are activated locally when a vessel is cut. This sequence of enzyme activation leading to fibrin formation is referred to as the *extrinsic system* because the stimulus for initiating the process is extrinsic to the blood vessels. The process can also be initiated by the exposure of blood to a nonendothelial surface (such as a dialyzer or vascular prosthesis). This activates a protein called *Factor XII* or *Hageman factor*. The activated form is called *Factor XIIa*. This series of enzymatic reactions proceeds through four steps, leading to activation of the extrinsic system at the level of the Factor X to Xa activation. This system of contact activation is referred to as the *intrinsic system*. These components of thrombogenesis are summarized in Figure 8-1.

Red blood cells, white blood cells, and other components of plasma are enmeshed in the platelet-fibrin aggregate as it grows at the site of the disrupted blood vessel. If the blood vessel is very small and the pressure is low (as in a capillary or venule), the platelet-fibrin plug fills the hole and stops the bleeding. The small vessel becomes occluded, and nutrient supply to the tissues continues through the process of collateral circulation. Blood that has leaked out before the platelet-fibrin plug stopped the bleeding becomes a large platelet-fibrin aggregate, or clot. If the injured blood vessel is large and the pressure is low (as in the inferior vena cava in our example), blood leaks out and forms clots but the platelet-fibrin aggregate adherent to the cut surfaces does not grow large enough to occlude the opening. When the pressure caused by the surrounding clot equals the pressure in the vein, bleeding stops and the platelet-fibrin plug (including the clot outside the vessel) seals the hole. If the vessel is large and the pressure is high (an artery), each systolic pulse pushes more blood through the hole into the surrounding clot and the clot may never reach a point where the pressure outside the vessel equals the arterial pressure, hence bleeding will continue despite the progressive formation of platelet-fibrin aggregate until it is stopped by local pressure, surgical intervention, or systemic hypotension equaling the clot pressure around the artery. In arteries the distance that the platelet-fibrin aggregate has to bridge is minimized by spasm of the smooth muscle in the arterial wall. Arterial spasm can prevent bleeding from large arteries for minutes or hours, if the vessel is totally transected. In our case bleeding capillaries, venules, and arterioles stopped bleeding within a minute through the operation of these mechanisms. Small arteries in the wall of the bowel and the muscle of the abdominal wall stopped bleeding when a combination of spasm and local tissue pressure facilitated the complete formation of the platelet-fibrin plugs. Blood from a 4-mm artery in the mesentery and blood exiting through the 1-cm hole in the wall of the vena cava drained freely into the peritoneum until the venous pressure was zero and the arterial pressure was 50 mm Hg. At this point the platelet-fibrin plug had sealed the holes, but only after 30% of the blood volume (1500 mL) had leaked into the peritoneum and clotted.

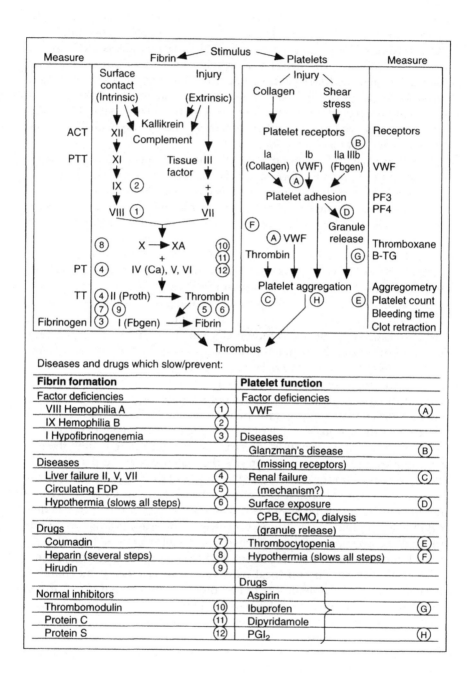

FIGURE 8-1. Summary of events in fibrin formation and platelet activation resulting in thrombosis. Tests to measure parts of the system are given on the sides and conditions that inhibit the system are shown as numbers and letters. (ACT = activated clotting time; B-TBG = B Thromboglobulin; Fbgen = fibrinogen; FDP = fibrin degradation products; PF = platelet factor; PT = prothrombin time; PTT = partial thromboplastin time; TT = thrombin time; VWF = von Willebrand factor.)

Tests of Thrombosis

Platelets

Platelets are made in the bone marrow by budding off of megakaryocytes. This process is stimulated by a hormone called *thrombopoietin*. Each platelet circulates for an average of 11 days, then is removed from the circulation in the fixed reticuloendothelial system, particularly in the spleen and liver. The balance of this generation and removal system results in approximately 300,000 platelets/mm^3 in circulating blood. As with most body systems, this number of platelets is five to ten times higher than the number actually needed for basal homeostasis and hemostasis. Thrombocytopenia itself may account for bleeding when the platelet count is less than 20 to 30,000/mm^3. Platelet function, although critically important, is notoriously difficult to measure. This is because almost every test of platelet function involves the inadvertent activation of the platelets before the test is done (in the process of drawing blood, injecting the blood into test devices, separating the platelets for analysis, and so on). For this reason, in vitro tests of platelet function are so insensitive as to be relatively useless for clinical purposes. These tests include aggregation in response to stimulation by adenosinediphosphates, epinephrine, or collagen and adherence to glass beads or other surfaces. It is possible to measure some of the products released from platelet granules, including platelet factor 4, thromboxane, and beta-thromboglobulin. However, these tests have little practical value aside from research applications to evaluate the effectiveness of platelet-inhibiting drugs. Platelets are important in facilitating the tightening of fibrin polymers long after a clot has formed, resulting in the process of clot retraction. Hence the absence of retraction when a clot is observed over the course of several hours indicates the possible presence of thrombocytopenia or thrombocytopathy. The only test of platelet function that is uniformly used is the bleeding time. In this test a small standardized incision is made in the finger or earlobe and the time it takes for the platelet-fibrin plug to form (that is, the cessation of bleeding) is measured. This test obviously crude and affected by so many factors that it is essentially useless in the critically ill patient.

Fibrin Formation

The various components of the fibrin formation sequence are measured by adding various activators to liquid blood or plasma and measuring the time it takes for the liquid to become gelatinous. All of these tests can be done on fresh unanticoagulated whole blood but are almost always done on plasma from blood that has been anticoagulated with a calcium chelator such as citrate or EDTA. This approach is taken for the purpose of standardization, because it is possible to compare results with those for a large pool of anticoagulated plasma from normal people, and also for convenience's sake, because a large number of fibrin formation tests can be run electively in a central laboratory. Because the plasma is anticoagulated with the calcium chelator, an excess of calcium is added at the same time as the activator to allow the fibrin formation reaction to run to completion. All of these tests are done in an incubator at 37°C. In the so-called screening tests, the time it takes for the liquid to become gelatinous is measured after the addition of thrombin (the thrombin time [TT]), standardized tissue thromboplastin (the prothrombin time [PT]), or kaolin and lipid from rabbit brain (the partial thromboplastin time [PTT] or accelerated partial thromboplastin time). In measuring the clotting time or activated clotting time (ACT), only the intrinsic system (factor XII) is activated by contact with glass or other silicates such as diatomaceous earth. Of course the intrinsic system is also activated in the other screening tests by the glass or plastic in which the test is done, but this reaction proceeds so much more slowly than that of the other activators that the intrinsic system is not significant in the final result of the TT, PT, or PTT. If the results of all these screening tests are normal (when compared with those for a pool of plasma from normal people), then it can be said that all of the fibrin formation sequence is normal.

If the results all of the screening tests are equally prolonged, the problem could be a lack of fibrinogen or the presence of an anticoagulant. If the TT is normal but the PT and PTT are prolonged, one or more factors above the level of fibrinogen are deficient. If the PT and TT are normal but the PTT or ACT is prolonged, there is most likely a deficiency of some factor above prothrombin in the sequence. In the latter case the specific factor deficiency is identified by repeating the PTT after various quantities of specific clotting factors are added to the test serum. In this fashion a specific factor defect can be both identified and quantitated, the latter expressed as the percentage of the normal amount of the factor involved. In addition to these tests that measure the time to fibrin formation, it is possible to separate and measure the actual amount of the various factors. Usually this is done for fibrinogen, the normal value of which is 300 mg/dL.

The screening tests are also used to titrate the anticoagulant dosage. Coumadin (sodium warfarin) inhibits prothrombin formation in the liver, and the level of prothrombin deficiency is estimated by the prolongation of the PT. Heparin combines with circulating antithrombin to form thrombin-antithrombin complexes, inhibiting fibrin formation at that level. Heparin also acts to inhibit other enzymatic reactions in the sequence. Consequently the heparin effect can be measured as a prolongation of the PTT or ACT. Although it is common practice to titrate heparin by the measured defect on PTT in plasma, the result can be quite misleading. Heparin interacts with red blood cells, white blood cells, and platelets, which in turn interact with the fibrin formation system, as previously described. For this reason, a person who is severely thrombocytopenic, for example, might be overanticoagulated if the plasma PTT alone is used as the gauge of the heparin effect. The best way to titrate the heparin dosage is to measure the whole blood ACT on fresh blood at the bedside or on chelator-anticoagulated blood in the central laboratory. Some laboratories report the heparin concentration in blood. This value is usually not a specific measurement of the heparin level but rather an estimate of the amount of heparin that would be required to achieve a given PTT in normal plasma. Because of the various factors just discussed, the actual amount of heparin in blood is irrelevant compared with the heparin effect, so the whole blood ACT remains the best way to regulate heparin dosage.

Tests of Fibrinolysis

Whenever fibrin is formed, plasminogen in the surrounding plasma is activated to become plasmin (fibrinolysin). This activation takes place relatively slowly and results in clot lysis beginning at approximately 12 hours at room temperature. There is no specific assay for plasmin. A test called the *euglobulin lysis time* can be done in which a standardized gelatinous fibrin clot is exposed to test plasma and the time required for liquefaction to occur is measured. This test is rarely necessary because the only clinical circumstance associated with isolated excess fibrinolysis is associated with the systemic absorption of urine, which is usually obvious for other reasons. In all other clinical circumstances in which fibrinolysis may be occurring, it is associated with previous or ongoing coagulation, so that the effect of fibrinolysis is most easily determined by measuring the amount of fibrin degradation products (FDPs) or fibrin split products in circulating blood. Normally there are no FDPs in circulating blood, so any evidence of these molecules is a sign of clot lysis with absorption of the breakdown products. Notice that clot lysis anywhere in the patient causes an elevation in the FDP levels. It is *not* an indication of *intra*vascular coagulation.

Bleeding and Clotting Abnormalities in Critical Care Patients

When an ICU patient is bleeding, we must decide whether the problem is simply related to vascular injury or caused by an underlying coagulopathy. Of course both may coexist, for example, in a patient with consumption coagulopathy who has a duodenal ulcer eroding into the gastroduodenal artery. Such a patient requires an emergency trip to the operating room to stop the bleeding while the coagulation status is also being restored to normal. As a rule of thumb, direct surgical intervention should be instituted whenever the blood loss in 24 hours or less is half the blood volume. In a patient with a severe coagulopathy, a modification of this rule of thumb is half the blood volume in 24 hours after the coagulopathy has been successfully treated. As noted in the case example, operation may be required before the coagulopathy has been successfully treated.

Major blood loss is treated with the infusion of clear fluids, colloid fluids, and blood products. Because platelets and clotting factors are consumed (or physically lost) in the process of bleeding and because the replacement fluids do not fully replace the lost materials, the most common abnormal coagulation finding associated with major bleeding is loss or consumption combined with dilution. In this situation there are usually blood clots in the patient that are being broken down and absorbed while the bleeding and dilution are going on. Consequently, blood tests will show a decrease in platelet numbers, an increase in the fibrin screening times, and significant levels of FDPs. The absorption of broken-down red blood cells may cause an elevated plasma hemoglobin level. This pattern of coagulation test results occurs with any type of bleeding treated by transfusion. It also occurs when clotting and lysis are taking place simultaneously at some point within the vascular system (localized intravascular coagulation), such as occurs in the setting of abruptio placenta or in massive hemangiomas (the Keisselbach-Merritt syndrome). The same test results are seen in disseminated intravascular coagulation [DIC]. DIC, which is essentially the same as thrombotic thrombocytopenic purpura, is exceptionally rare compared with the test pattern that occurs as the consequence of internal bleeding and transfusion, or localized intravascular coagulation. DIC can occur when Factor XII is activated by antigen-antibody complexes, bacterial endotoxin, or certain toxins such as snake venom. The term *DIC* is often used incorrectly. It is purely a pathologist's diagnosis and is based on the finding of intravascular thrombosis in multiple tissues. *Consumption coagulopathy with fibrinolysis* is a much better term for this particular pattern of coagulation abnormality. These patterns of laboratory test findings are summarized in Table 8-1.

Specific factor defects can be identified by a combination of screening tests and specific factor tests. A deficiency of fibrinogen or of any of the protein

TABLE 8-1. Typical Patterns of Coagulopathy*

	Platelet count	Bleeding time	Fibrinogen	PTT or ACT	PT	TT	FDP
External bleeding and transfusion	↓	↑	↓	↑	↑	↑	0
Internal bleeding and transfusion (very common)	↓	↑	↓	↑	↑	↑	↑
DIC (very rare)	↓	↑	↓	↑	↑	↑	↑
Thrombocytopenia	↓	↑	N	N	N	N	0
Thrombocytopathia	N	↑	N	N	N	N	0
Liver failure	N	↑	↓	↑	↑	↑	0
Hemophilia	N	N	N	↑	N	N	0
Coumadin	N	N	N	↑	↑	N	0
Heparin	N	N	N	↑	N	↑	0
von Willebrand's disease	N	↑	N	N↑	N	N	0
Fibrinolysis	N	N	N	↑	↑	↑	↑
PRBC and saline	0	—	N	N	N	N	0
Frozen plasma	0	—	N	N	N	N	0
Platelets	↑	—	N	N	N	N	0

*Abnormal coagulation test results associated with various clinical conditions. Notice that the pattern for internal bleeding associated with transfusion and DIC is the same.

ACT = activated clotting time; DIC = disseminated intravascular coagulation; FDP = fibrin degradation products; N = normal; PRBC = packed red blood cells; PT = prothrombin time; PTT = partial thromboplastin time; TT = thrombin time; ↑ = increased; ↓ = decreased; 0 = none.

coagulation factors can be treated with fresh frozen plasma, given in quantities sufficient to return the screening test results to normal. Reconstituted cryoprecipitate is a more concentrated solution of plasma proteins, which is rich in clotting factors. It is more complicated to prepare than plasma and therefore more expensive. Cryoprecipitate is used when existing hypervolemia makes the infusion of plasma dangerous. Specific coagulation factors are available for specific factor deficiencies, such as antihemophilic globulin (concentrated Factor VIII) for hemophilia A.

Platelet-rich plasma is given when bleeding is caused by thrombocytopenia or when platelet dysfunction is suspected. Platelet transfusion is indicated when the platelet count is less than $30,000/m^3$ or when the bleeding time is grossly prolonged. The latter is usually not evaluated by a standardized lancet incision, but more commonly by simply observing the nature of bleeding after the levels of other coagulation factors have been returned to normal. Platelet-rich plasma typically contains 400,000 to 600,000 platelets/mm^3 in 50 mL of plasma. If the blood volume is 5 L and if platelet loss has stopped, the infusion of 50 mL of plasma containing 600,000 platelets /mm^3 will raise the actual platelet count by $6000/mm^3$. It is common practice to give six units of platelet-rich plasma at a time, which should raise the platelet count by $36,000/mm^3$ (given the above assumption). Platelets that have been separated from donor blood, stored, then transfused are less active than normal platelets and have a much shorter half-life. Consequently a patient who is being transfused with platelets for the treatment of thrombocytopenia will need progressively larger amounts of platelets transfused to maintain a given peripheral blood platelet count. Finally, it is very important to note that neither platelets nor the enzymes of the fibrin formation cascade work well when cold. Even moderate hypothermia (34° to 36°C) will result in a severe coagulopathy. In the setting of bleeding and transfusion in a paralyzed or comatose patient, it is common to find temperatures in the range of 33° to 34°C. No amount of fresh frozen plasma or platelets will stop bleeding in such a patient. Remember that the coagulation tests are done at 37°C, so coagulation test results may appear to be perfectly normal in a patient who actually has hypothermic coagulopathy. Our algorithm for the evaluation and management of bleeding is shown in Figure 8-2.

In our case example, we expect to find clot and liquid blood in the abdomen and retroperitoneum. We avoid dislodging retroperitoneal clot until we can control aortic and caval inflow and outflow. We are careful to maintain the core temperature at more than 36°C. If red blood cell replacement exceeds one blood volume (eight to ten units of packed red blood cells), we give some fresh frozen plasma and six units of platelets to replace the presumed (or measured) consumption and loss. One to two days after operation we expect to find moderate thrombocytopenia; a slight elevation in the PT, PTT, and TT; and moderately high levels of FDPs. The intern calls this DIC, but he is incorrect.

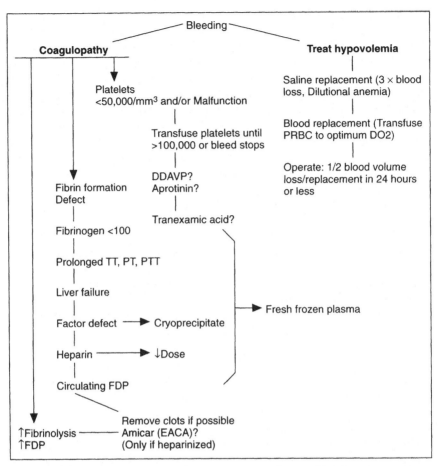

FIGURE 8-2. An algorithm for the management of active bleeding. Prevention of hypothermia is an essential step. (DDAVP = desmopressin acetate; EACA = epsilon-aminocaproic acid; FDP = fibrin degradation products; PT = prothrombin time; PTT = partial thromboplastin time; TT = thrombin time.)

Inflammation

Whenever endothelium is injured or denuded from the underlying basement membrane, circulating white blood cells adhere to the exposed collagen. The most prominent of these is the neutrophil, but lymphocytes, mast cells, and monocytes stop at the site of injury and expel their cytoplasmic contents such as histamine, lysosomal enzymes, and superoxide and hydroxyl radicals. Oxides combine instantly with chloride and then adjacent proteins to form chloramines. These activated leukocytes also produce a series of small peptides called *interleukin cytokines* because their primary function is to provide a means of communication to other white blood cells.

The net result of this local slurry of unusual chemicals is an increase in capillary permeability, permitting fluid and intact white blood cells to go through the capillary walls to the interstitial fluid. The change in capillary permeability is not enough to result in bleeding or even the loss of large proteins (in most cases), but does cause extravasation of water, electrolytes, and other molecules up to the size of albumin molecules. The fluid itself is detectable as edema. The neutrophils phagocytose bits of red blood cells and platelets when the clot lyses. Local vasodilatation results in increased blood flow, causing warmth and redness. The systemic absorption of interleukins may result in fever. These signs of inflammation are usually minimal if the injury is not associated with bacterial contamination, the presence of foreign bodies, or tissue necrosis. T lymphocytes that initiate the antibody response cycle, monocytes that generate the proteolytic cytokine tumor necrosis factor (TNF), and complement that speeds up all these processes are "alerted" by the family of interleukins but are not activated unless there is antigenic material at the site of injury. Some of these events are summarized in Figure 8-3.

In our case example the clots in the abdomen and all of the tissues that have been opened are contaminated with feces, which includes all manner of animal and vegetable debris and billions of bacteria. The grossly visible particles have been removed at operation, and the free-floating bacteria have been diluted by irrigation and killed with topical antiseptics. Antibiotics are given intravenously with the hope that they will permeate the edema fluid, but despite all these measures we know that the tissues in the peritoneum, vena caval wall, stab wound, and surgical incision are loaded with a wide variety of bacteria. These bacteria are in a medium rich in protein and sugar at a temperature of 37°C. They grow as fast as they can, producing endotoxin and exotoxin or just more bacteria, depending on the species. The surface antigens and toxins speed up every aspect of the inflammatory process. Now T cells carry the antigens to local lymph nodes, where antibody-producing B cells are activated. Monocytes and fixed tissue histiocytes generate enough TNF to cause systemic proteolysis. Neutrophils produce enough interleukins to be absorbed systemically, causing fever and hypermetabolism. Activated complement, histamine, and other mediators may cause generalized capillary permeability. Bacteria are phagocytosed, killed, and expectorated by neutrophils, resulting in a turbid fluid called *pus* that further stimulates and accelerates the process of inflammation. Now there is more than inflammation, there is inflammation with infection. The same level of inflammation occurs at the interface between necrotic but sterile tissue and healthy tissue and is exaggerated when necrosis is caused by a toxin or enzyme, as in the setting of pancreatitis or snake bite.

Local inflammation results in a remarkable example of neoplasia at the interface between healthy tissue and infected (or necrotic) tissue. This interface is referred to as *granulation tissue* and is actually an active neoplasm that is several millimeters thick. This remarkable tissue is primarily composed

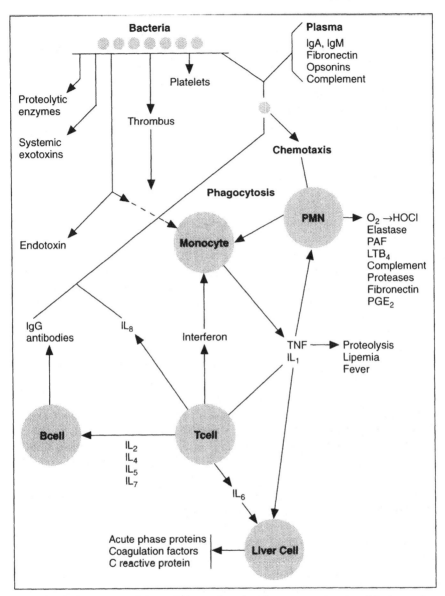

FIGURE 8-3. Some of the cellular and molecular events stimulated by bacteria in tissues. (IL = interleukin; LTB4 = leukotriene B_4; PAF = platelet-activating factor; PGE_2 = prostaglandin E_2; PMN = polymorphonuclear leukocytes.)

of capillaries, bringing a nonstop supply of new leukocytes to the infection. Meanwhile fibroblasts are laying down a barrier of collagen between the healthy tissue and the granulation tissue, preventing the further invasion of growing bacteria. In this fashion the infection is partially isolated from the rest of the body. The pus is said to be "walled off," and the entire process is described as an *abscess*.

What happens to the abscess is determined by the balance between the number and type of bacteria and the number and activity of leukocytes. If the white blood cells predominate, the fluid will be rendered sterile and eventually resorbed. If the bacteria predominate, toxins and intact bacteria will be absorbed into the capillaries, causing septicemia and the dysfunction of other organs. If the patient survives this continuing septicemia, the nonstop production of pus will push aside the tissues that offer the least resistance, ultimately resulting in the abscess appearing in the subcutaneous tissue ("pointing") and ultimately leading to external drainage through the skin. When the abscess is externally drained (either by spontaneous rupture or placement of a drainage tube), or if the abscess is small and the fluid is rendered sterile and resorbed, the neoplastic granulation tissue slowly but miraculously disappears, leaving only the empty space surrounded by a thick collagen scar. Over a period of months the collagen scar contracts as the polymer cross-links more and more, obliterating the space and leaving only a little scar tissue.

An interesting experiment of nature illustrates the differences between bacterial-infected inflammation and the systemic symptoms produced simply by ongoing inflammation. Patients with an expanding abscess (pus under pressure) suffer intermittent fever, rigors, metastatic infection, bacteremia, leukocytosis, tachycardia, hypermetabolism, ileus, and proteolysis. These are also signs and symptoms of systemic or non–walled-off infection such as meningococcemia, streptococcal septicemia, or fresh peritonitis. After the abscess has been drained, fever, rigors, bacteremia, metastatic infection, hypermetabolism, and tachycardia disappear in a day or two. Leukocytosis and proteolysis continue, particularly if the granulation tissue wall is thick. These symptoms are typical of isolated monocyte and neutrophil activation and continue until the granulation tissue has healed and resolved. If an abdominal abscess is drained externally but granulation tissue is continually activated by an enteric fistula or smoldering pancreatitis, the process can continue for months. With a drained infection, ileus resolves and it is possible to resume enteric feeding, but cachexia, weakness, and catabolism persist until the granulation tissue has been resorbed and healed.

If the organ affected by extensive inflammation with bacteria or tissue necrosis malfunctions during any of these phases, then death or morbidity may result. For example, if the primary problem is in the lung, brain, or myocardium, acute or chronic dysfunction may be irreversible.

One aspect of inflammation of major importance to ICU patients is the normal interfaces between bacterial colonization and internal tissues. These interfaces occur at the skin, the conjunctivae, the oropharyngeal mucosa, the respiratory mucosa, the vagina, and the entire gastrointestinal tract, particularly the ileum and colon. The skin is transgressed by surgical incisions and a variety of tubes and catheters placed for monitoring, blood sampling, and drainage. Any organisms on the skin can and will find their way along these catheters, drains, and incisions. Bacteria normally present in the eyes, nose, and mouth proliferate and may cause local infection, particularly in the eyes and sinuses. The respiratory tract is normally sterile below the level of the vocal cords, but the aspiration of oral fluids, with or without endotracheal intubation, causes the lower airway to be contaminated with mouth organisms. Pneumonitis, sinusitis, parotitis, and infection of the fibrin sheath surrounding intervascular catheters are all examples of nosocomial or hospital-acquired infections. All the principles of infected inflammation previously listed apply to these circumstances. Even more interesting is the barrier between the grossly contaminated intestinal tract and the portal blood circulation. Diseases that cause damage to the lower intestinal epithelium, such as colitis, diverticulitis, protozoan colitis, salmonellosis, shigellosis, and typhoid fever, often lead to the direct absorption of bacteria and bacterial toxins into the portal venous blood. These bacteria may be cleared by the reticuloendothelial system in the liver, or infection may result in liver abscess or in systemic bacteremia and septicemia. Other conditions which occur in critically ill patients, such as shock, intestinal ischemia, and the intestinal atrophy associated with a lack of enteral feeding, result in a change in the permeability of the intestinal mucosa that may invite the absorption of exotoxins and endotoxins (if not live bacteria), causing the septic syndrome. This may occur even though bacteria are not cultured from the bloodstream. This phenomenon can be produced experimentally in animals and is certainly likely to occur in human subjects. Some investigators are convinced that this always occurs, referring to the gut as the "motor" of the systemic inflammatory response syndrome (SIRS) and the source of multisystem organ failure. However, this is certainly not a universal phenomenon, and efforts to prevent it are not always effective. Nonetheless, it makes good sense to clear the intestine of gross feces in critically ill patients, provide some nonabsorbable intestinal antibiotic protection or antisepsis, and prevent intestinal mucosal atrophy as much as possible by providing some enteric feeding. The amino acid glutamine seems to be particularly important in this regard.

Tests of Inflammation and Infection

After the vital signs are evaluated, the white blood cell and differential counts are the starting point for the evaluation of infection. Inflammation is usually associated with leukocytosis and an increased percentage of neutrophils, but very severe infection or necrosis can deplete the number of circulating leukocytes faster than they are replaced from the bone marrow, resulting in neutropenia. A very detailed differential count identifying specific categories of lymphocytes is done through a process known as *flow cytometry*. In this process, T cells, B cells, and a variety of subclassifications of these cells can be identified and quantitated. This is particularly important in the evaluation of patients treated with immunosuppressive drugs specifically designed to deplete subsets of the T-cell population. It is also important in patients with the acquired immune deficiency syndrome (AIDS). In this condition the extent of immunosuppression can be evaluated by the CD4/CD8 ratio (normal, 1.8 to 2.2).

Tests of white blood cell function are available for research purposes but are rarely used clinically, probably because these tests generally require separating white blood cells into various types, then incubating them with bacteria, dyes, or other chemicals to determine the status of phagocytosis, intracellular bacterial killing, and chemotaxis. Aside from their complexity and expense, another reason for why these tests are not used clinically is because there is as yet no practical means of improving white blood cell or reticuloendothelial function if it is found to be deficient. The only test of white blood cell function that has found widespread application is the test of skin reactivity of cell-mediated immunity introduced by the McGill surgical research group for use in critically ill patients. In this test, five common antigens are inoculated into the deep dermis and the inflammatory response is measured 24 and 48 hours later. This is exactly like a tuberculin skin test, and in fact tuberculin is one of the five antigens, along with trichophyton, streptococcal antigen, *Candida*, and mumps antigens. These antigens were picked because it was assumed that most adults would have developed antibodies to most of them. The development of a local wheal, induration, and erythema in at least three antigen sites is considered a normal response. No response at all is considered a sign of anergy. Although this is a test of cell-mediated immunity, it is used as a test of the entire inflammatory response, with particular emphasis on the ability of the patient to respond to bacterial infection. Anergy is associated with malnutrition, acute illness, cancer, and an increased incidence of bacterial infection and mortality in the setting of critical illness or after major operations. If skin test reactivity converts from an anergic to reactive status after nutritional treatment or recovery from critical illness, mortality is reduced. Because there are other simpler methods of evaluating the acute nutritional status in critically ill patients, skin test reactivity is not generally used in critically ill patients. However, it is helpful in evaluating patients who are being considered for major elective operations to determine whether preoperative nutritional treatment is likely to be beneficial.

Like the circulating white blood cells, the fixed-tissue reticuloendothelial system can be evaluated by the clearance of injected particles or substances from the blood. However, these tests are generally reserved for research studies because there is no specific way to treat reticuloendothelial system malfunction if it is detected.

Measurement of the chemical products of inflammation is moving from the arena of clinical research to that of clinical practice. All of the several interleukins, leukotrienes, adhesion molecules, and products of abnormal oxidative metabolism can be measured in blood, sputum, and other body fluids. Of all these molecules, measurement of TNF is emerging as the most important one for practical clinical testing because TNF is a final common denominator for all types of inflammation and because it has significant physiologic effects. However, to date measurement of these mediators has not been found to either predict or even correlate with the outcome from inflammatory syndromes.

Measurement of bacteria by culture and antibiotic sensitivity is the mainstay in the planning of antibiotic or antiseptic treatment. Gram's staining is useful for the immediate general classification of bacterial infection, and qualitative and quantitative cultures can identify specific organisms. The choice of antibiotic drugs is initially based on a guess as to the most likely cause of infection, and drug choices are modified once the culture and antibiotic sensitivities are known (Figure 8-4).

There is an assay for the lipopolysaccharide endotoxin produced by most gram-negative organisms, but it is not often used in clinical practice. This assay is called the *limulus assay* because the reagent is blood from the horseshoe crab (*Limulus*). The assay consists of a color change in the copper-based pigment of *Limulus* blood induced by endotoxin. Because bacterial endotoxin appears to have physiologic effects mediated only by TNF stimulation and release, direct measurement of TNF is replacing endotoxin measurement, even in research studies. Some specific toxins elaborated by bacteria are useful for clinical tests, particularly the identification of *Clostridium difficile* toxin in the evaluation of infectious diarrhea.

Applications in Critical Care Patients

The primary treatment for inflammation and infection is external drainage, if possible. For the treatment of a symptomatic sterile inflammation this may require the removal of necrotic or ischemic tissue, such as burn eschar, or drainage of the inflammatory source, such as of the lesser omental space in the setting of acute pancreatitis. For the treatment of infectious inflammation this may require removing the source of infection, such as endocarditis affecting a tricuspid valve, or draining the lesion causing the localized infection, such as an empyema or abscess. If the infection is not localized or is not amenable to resection or surgical drainage, as in bacterial pneumonitis, then antibiotics become the mainstay of treatment. It is important to keep these priorities in order, however. No amount of antibiotics will sterilize a pus-filled

Critical Care Physiology

Family	Antibiotic	IV Dose	Relative Cost/d	Staphcoag–	Staphcoag+	MRS	Strep A, B	Enterococcus	H flu	Bacteroides	Clostridium p	Common Gm–	Enterobacter	Pseudomonas	Serratia	Citrobacter	Acinetobacter
Penicillins	Pen G	2 mill q 4	10	●			●	o			●						
	Methicillin	1 gm q 4	30	o	●												
	Oxacillin	1 gm q 4	60	o	o												
Other Gm+	Vancomycin	.5 gm q 6	32	o	o	●	o	o									
Aminopens	Ampicillin	.5 gm q 6	16	o			o	●	●		o						
	Aztreonam	1 gm q 8	30									o		o	o		
Combinations	(Timentin)	3 gm q 4	54	o	o					o	o	o	o		o		o
	(Unasyn)	1 gm q 6	20	o	o					o	●	o					
	(Primaxin)	.5 gm qp 4	90	o	o					o	o	o	o	o	o	o	o
Macrolide	Erythromycin	.25 gm q 4	30	o	o		o										
Cephalosporin I	Cephalothin (Keflin)	1 gm q 4	18														
	Cefazolin (Kefzol)	1 gm q 6	24	o	o						o	o	●				
II	Cefotetan (Cefotan)	1 gm q 12	20														
	Cefuroxime (Zinacef)	1 gm q 8	24	o	o						o	o	o		o		
III	Cefotaxime (Claforan)	1 gm q 8	30														
	Ceftriaxone (Rocephin)	1 gm q 12	60	o	o				o			o	o			●	●
	Ceftazidine (Fortaz)	1 gm q 8	42														
Anti Ps III	Cefoperazone (Cefobid)	1 gm q 8	30	o	o							o	o	●	●	●	
Aminoglycosides	Gentamycin	.08 gm q 8	6	o	o	o		o				●	●	●	o	o	●
	Tobramycin	.08 gm q 8	21	o	o	o		o				o	o	o	o	o	o
	Amikacin	.5 gm q 8	120	o	o	o		o				o	o	o	o	o	o
Other Gm–	Metronidazole (Flagyl)	.5 gm q 6	48							●	o						
	Trimethoprim sulfa (Bactrim)	.25 gm q 6	88	o	o							o	o		o		
	Clindamycin	.6 gm q 8	33							o	o						
	Chloramphenicol	1 gm q 6	16	o	o		o	o	o	o	o	o					
Quinoline	Floxin	.4 gm q 8	9	o	o	o		o				●	●	o	o	o	o
Antifungal	Amphotericin B	.05 gm q 24	27														
	Fluconazole	.2 gm q 12	20														
Antiviral	Acyclovir	1 gm q 8	240														
	Gancyclovir	.5 gm q 12	240														

o = Usually sensitive
● = Drug(s) of choice

FIGURE 8-4. Typical sensitivities, dosage, and relative cost (in dollars) of common antibiotics. The dosage and cost are those for typical parenteral doses used in the treatment of severe infection. The drug of choice indicated for specific species is the author's preference. (Clostridium p = *Clostridium perfringens;* Gm+ = gram-positive; Gm– = gram-negative; H flu = *Haemophilus influenzae;* MRS = methicillin-resistant *Staphylococcus aureus.*)

gallbladder, pleural space, subcutaneous abscess, or necrotizing fasciitis. If antibiotics are necessary for treatment, the choice is determined initially by an informed guess regarding the species of bacteria involved, then a change in antibiotics if necessary when the specific species and antibiotic sensitivity have been identified. A list of common bacteria and commonly used antibiotics is shown in Figure 8-4.

Multiple-Organ Failure and the SIRS

Every patient in the ICU is there because of an inflammatory or infectious disease, or is at risk for infection. Much of ICU monitoring is intended to detect the earliest stages of inflammation or infection and to measure the response to treatment. Although many assays of the inflammatory process are available, as already mentioned, current practice depends on simple assessments such as temperature, the white blood cell count, the differential count, the pulse rate, cultures, and of course physical examination. This is appropriate because it is the response to inflammation and infection that we wish to assess, not the mediators themselves. For example, suppose we find that blood levels of TNF and interleukin-6 and interleukin-8 are increasing while a patient is showing clinical signs of significant improvement from an episode of pancreatitis or bacterial pneumonitis. We might worry about a pancreatic abscess or empyema, but we had that worry anyway. We would not change our treatment on the basis of these measured levels of mediators, just as we would not change an insulin dose on the basis of measured levels of serum insulin when the blood glucose level is normal. However, the measurement of mediator levels and the treatment instituted on the basis of these measurements will undoubtedly become an important part of the management of the systemic inflammatory response syndrome (SIRS).

A common problem in any ICU is the patient who has fever, leukocytosis, tachycardia, an elevated metabolic rate, and protein catabolism—all the signs of bacterial infection—but whose culture results are negative and in whom no source of infection can be found. These patients often have an abnormal increase in capillary permeability, which may lead to specific organ dysfunction in the lungs (adult or acute respiratory distress syndrome [ARDS]), in the kidney (acute tubular necrosis), the gut (lack of peristalsis or ileus), the heart (myocardial edema resulting in decreased contractility or "myocardial depression"), the liver (cholestatic jaundice), or the brain (confusion, disorientation, stupor, and coma, known collectively as *metabolic encephalopathy*). These conditions are often referred to as being septoid, or as *ARDS, multiple-organ failure*, or most recently as the *SIRS*. *SIRS* is the most appropriate term because the manifestations all result from systemic responses apparently caused by cells and mediators that are usually activated locally. If a primary source of infection or inflammation can be identified and treated, the distant organ manifestations of the syndrome usually disappear promptly—adding further evidence supporting the theory that multiple-organ failure or SIRS is driven by a local inflammation or infection. As discussed earlier, the intestine is often referred to as the "motor" of SIRS. This is certainly true in cases of severe primary intestinal disease, such as toxic megacolon and may well be true in other cases of critical illness. It makes sense to evacuate and attempt to sterilize the colon and lower small intestine in those patients whose primary problem is pneumonia, trauma, liver failure, or hemorrhagic shock.

Another application spawned by our knowledge of the physiology of inflammation is the use of drugs designed to inhibit specific components of the inflammatory response in an attempt to decrease the incidence and severity of the effect of systemic inflammatory mediators and cells. For example, the generalized inhibition of inflammation brought about by huge doses of corticosteroids has been advocated in the treatment of sepsis, septic shock, generic ARDS, pancreatitis, burns, and pulmonary bone marrow (fat) embolism. The latter is an excellent example because it is a pure sterile inflammation occurring at the level of the lung capillaries. In an experimental preparation, large doses of steroids have been observed to prevent the capillary leakage associated with fat embolism when given before the event and even after the event when given within the first hour or so. Steroids given hours after a fat embolism forms blunt the pulmonary response but inhibit the total inflammatory response so completely that the risk of bacterial infection and poor healing overrides any potential benefit conferred by the agents. This same problem has led to the conclusion that steroids are more harmful than helpful in the treatment of any of the conditions just listed. As new inhibitors of the inflammatory response reach clinical trials, we must carefully read the papers describing them, with the concern that preventing ARDS, for example, may be possible but may lead to other complications, such that the overall morbidity and mortality are not ultimately affected.

Nosocomial infection is a major problem in ICU patients. Infection of intravascular catheters and bacterial pneumonia are the most common nosocomial infections, followed by *Clostridium difficile* colitis, acalculous cholecystitis, urinary tract infection, and closed-space infections such as sinusitis and otitis. Prophylaxis is obviously the best approach to preventing this problem and includes thorough cleaning and the application of antiseptic agents to transcutaneous catheters as well as oropharyngeal hygiene in intubated patients. The most important step in preventing infection in transcutaneous catheters is frequent physical cleaning with soap and water. It is a myth that patients with transcutaneous tubes or catheters should not bathe or shower, or that fresh incisions or catheters should always be kept dry. On the contrary, bathing, showering, or local cleaning is the best way to prevent catheter or drain tract infection. The application of antiseptic ointment to the skin site and the use of antiseptic-impregnated catheters can be used as adjuncts to local cleaning.

Similar principles apply to the airway. Nosocomial pneumonia is clearly related to the tracking of oropharyngeal organisms along the endotracheal tube. The number and type of bacteria finding their way into the lower airway are best minimized by keeping the oropharynx clean by frequent mouth care and lavage, and the application of topical antiseptics in the mouth. This is difficult in the patient with an oral endotracheal tube and impossible in the patient with a nasotracheal tube because the nasal and sinus mucosa is inaccessible on the side where the tube has been placed. In addition to the mouth organisms, bacteria and yeast normally killed in the stomach by the stomach acid may proliferate and appear in the mouth as regurgitated fluid in patients who have been rendered achlorhydric by histamine blockers or antacid drugs. For this reason the incidence of nosocomial pneumonia is much higher in patients who maintain a neutral gastric pH. Steps that can be taken in the ICU to prevent nosocomial pneumonia in intubated patients include careful and frequent oral hygiene, the application of topical antiseptics or nonabsorbable antibiotics in the mouth and throat, and the avoidance of gastric acid neutralization unless it is absolutely necessary. (The use of a gastric-coating agent such as Carafate [sucralfate] is as effective as antacids in preventing stress bleeding and minimizes the risk of nosocomial pneumonia in intubated patients.) Rather than, or in addition to, this emphasis on oropharyngeal decontamination is a use of tracheostomy rather than endotracheal intubation for patients who are going to need mechanical ventilation for more than a few days. The use of a tracheostomy for the management of patients in respiratory failure (which we prefer) assumes that tracheostomy can be done routinely without complications.

Management of the immunosuppressed patient follows all the principles just outlined. If an immunosuppressed patient has a life-threatening infection, stopping the immunosuppression regimen should be considered. For example, a patient with a kidney or pancreas transplant can be returned to mechanical or pharmacologic treatment if the grafts are rejected because of stopping the immunosuppression regimen. This is not true of a liver, heart, or lung transplant recipient. A patient who is immunosuppressed because of chemotherapy for cancer and who is dying of infection is in a lethal dilemma, the "solution" to which relates more to the mode of dying rather than to the chances of survival. The immunosuppressive drugs used for transplant patients (aside from steroids) are designed to inhibit lymphocyte function primarily, so that infections in these patients are usually viral or protozoan. The same applies to patients with primary lymphocyte disorders such as AIDS. Patients who are immunosuppressed because of malnutrition or bone marrow toxicity are subject to both viral and bacterial infections. Granulocyte transfusions and generic bone marrow stimulants have not proved practical in the presence of severe infection.

In our case example, we administer oxacillin and gentamycin empirically before, during, and 2 days after operation. We irrigate the abdomen with 4 liters of Dakin's solution before closing the peritoneum. We do not culture the feces in the abdomen. We close the fascia and leave a Dakin's pack in the open subcutaneous space. We do a colostomy to eliminate the risk of colon leak. Postoperatively we expect fever, leukocytosis, ileus, and hypermetabolism to last for the first 4 to 5 days. We start full parenteral nutrition on postoperative day 1 and gastric feeding with a high protein formula on day 2.

Healing and Fibrosis

The final stage of the host defense system process is healing, which is characterized by fibrosis, or collagen scar formation. This begins 3 to 4 days after the initial injury as fibroblasts begin to secrete collagen precursors and continues for a year or more, finally resulting in an avascular contracted collagen scar. The healing process is essentially the same whether the injury is a sterile surgical incision, an infected abscess wall, or pulmonary parenchymal destruction stemming from bacterial or viral infection. The first event in wound healing is coagulation, as the injured tissues are "glued together" with fibrin. Fibrin formation seals the area from external bacterial contamination and maintains the site of injury closed unless the fibrin is dissolved by bacterial infection or the edges are physically pulled apart. The tensile strength of the fibrin bond is very low, so that it takes minimal force to pull the fibrin-bonded area open. The next event in healing (after the neutrophil and monocyte inflammatory process begins, as described earlier) is the activation of fibroblasts to begin to produce elementary collagen known as *tropocollagen*. At the same time, new capillaries are formed that bridge the fibrin-sealed injury from one side to the other. By 5 to 7 days after injury the collagen molecules have begun to polymerize and the entire area is supplied by a new and rich capillary network. At 7 days all the elements of healing are well in place and functional. The tensile strength, however, is only about 10% of that of similar normal tissue (skin, bowel, muscle, and fascia). Fibroblasts continue to form collagen, and the collagen cross-links into thick polymer bundles. Both collagen formation and collagen lysis occur in actively healing wounds. The total collagen content (usually measured as the amount of hydroxyproline, the predominant amino acid in collagen) reaches a maximum 3 to 5 weeks after injury. If the injury includes a skin wound, this process is easily visible as an elevated indurated, purple (because of the capillary vascularity), epithelium-covered early scar. At 6 weeks the tensile strength is approximately 60% of that of normal tissue and the entire healing area has a dense new capillary network. This is why reoperation in a healing area 1 to 2 months after injury or operation is notoriously difficult.

Over the next 12 months the collagen becomes more and more heavily cross-linked, eventually closing off the capillary network and pulling the collagen strands tightly together, resulting in wound contracture. Approximately 12 months after injury, only a small collagen ball or band remains in the area of the injury. The tensile strength is then approximately 70% of

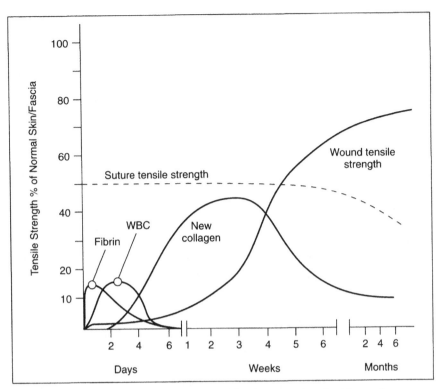

FIGURE 8-5. Chemical events in wound healing correlated with tensile strength. Typical relative values for skin and fascia are shown. Normal = 100%.

normal. At 1 year the skin wound should appear as a fine white line with no capillary blush. The sequence of events in healing is shown in Figure 8-5.

Healing is inhibited by infection, foreign body reaction, radiation, corticosteroids, scurvy, uremia, liver failure, and diabetes mellitus.

Tests of Healing in Fibrosis

Aside from laboratory and clinical research studies, there are no routine clinical tests to evaluate the healing process. In a critically ill patient a deficiency of healing is usually made obvious by the presence of continuing infection and draining wounds, and by fistula formation. Excess healing with the obliteration of normal tissue structure by fibrosis is most commonly seen as a total obliteration of lung architecture in response to generalized lung inflammation in the setting of ARDS or lung infectious diseases. The same process can also account for the obliteration of liver structure and function after severe or repeated liver injury (cirrhosis) or for bilateral renal cortical necrosis and fibrosis that occur after acute renal failure.

Application to Critically Ill Patients

One of the remarkable aspects of metabolic physiology is that inflammation proceeds to healing and fibrosis in critically ill patients, even in the face of protein catabolism and a negative energy or caloric balance, and despite the influence of systemic illness and a variety of drugs. The wound is said to act as a parasite on normal body protein metabolism, and indeed it is. Sterile wounds and sterile tissue injury in the lung, liver, and other organs will heal even in severely cachetic or debilitated patients. If the area of injury exists because of infection, as in necrotizing pneumonia, or becomes secondarily infected, as in a pancreatic abscess, collagen is often destroyed more quickly than it is laid down, the neovasculature may thrombose under the influence of bacterial toxins or other procoagulants, and healing is delayed or disrupted. At the interface between infected and healthy tissue, granulation tissue forms rapidly, but if the margins of the area of injury are separated by a collection of pus, tissue closure cannot occur. Once the pus is drained externally, coughed up, or resorbed, the scar formation continues, with the collagen in the walls of the injured area eventually contracting to obliterate the space altogether. This is the process that results in the formation of pneumatoceles and "honeycombing" after severe pulmonary infection, and also the process that explains the disappearance of pneumatoceles during the 6 to 12 months after clearance of the infection.

ICU patients are often treated with medications that impede healing, particularly corticosteroids. Steroids act to impede wound healing by inhibiting the inflammatory process in general and by causing protein catabolism. Collagen formation and tensile strength are significantly impeded in patients treated with corticosteroids (or patients with diabetes mellitus). An immunosuppressive state does not interfere with wound healing, except for increasing the susceptibility to bacterial infection. There is some experimental evidence to indicate that topical or systemic treatment with large quantities of vitamin A promotes normal healing in patients being treated with corticosteroid drugs. Aside from this, and despite the investigation of many materials, there is as yet no way to speed up healing in an injured area.

The management of open wounds is a common problem in the surgical ICU and merits some specific discussion. *Open wounds* usually refers to surgical incisions or injuries that have been closed to promote healing at the level of the underlying muscle fascia, but the subcutaneous tissue and skin are left open. Because the most common wound infections are localized to the subcutaneous fat, by leaving wounds open (or opening infected wounds) the potential for abscess formation is automatically eliminated. Fat, fascia, and skin edges are covered by dressings. The wound–dressing or wound–air interface acts as a foreign body stimulus, and the inflammatory process proceeds rapidly, leading to the visible formation of granulation tissue within a few days after the injury. Within a week or two the entire exposed open wound is covered by red, velvety granulation tissue, which acts as a good barrier to bacterial invasion (although not as good as intact skin), and provides a richly vascularized bed that can be skin grafted. Such a wound is allowed to heal by contracture and the migration of skin epithelium over the surface or is pulled together in apposition with the hope of healing (so-called delayed primary closure). Dealing with open wounds introduces one other factor that inhibits healing—the drying out or desiccation of the tissues. The best way to manage an open wound is quite simple: Keep it wet, keep it clean, and keep it as sterile as possible. Keeping the wound wet prevents desiccation and microthrombosis at the surface of the granulation tissue. The wound can be maintained wet with an isosmotic solution such as saline or with a hydrophilic, water-soluble cream. (The wound can also be kept wet with a hydrophobic ointment, but this may have the added effect of a foreign body and result in maceration of the wound.) Aside from the positive effects on wound healing, a wet wound is not painful. Keeping the wound clean entails daily inspection and physical debridement of the necrotic, infected, or desiccated areas. Debridement can be done by sharp surgical debridement or by the topical application of collagenase or other proteolytic enzymes. The process of packing a wound with gauze to remove debris when the adherent gauze is removed is painful, ineffective, and unnecessary in the management of open wounds. The purpose of packing is simply to keep the wound edges open so that the tissue can drain and ultimately heal before the skin heals. A secondary purpose of packs is to hold moisture and antiseptic drugs at the actively granulating surface.

The third objective is to keep the wound as sterile as possible. This is best accomplished by physical washing in a tub or shower or at the bedside. After thorough washing, if there is no necrotic tissue in the wound, bacterial counts are decreased to the first or second power and the wound is close to being sterile. Any bacteria present will grow following a typical bacterial logarithmic growth curve, so that bacterial counts over 10^5 per gram of tissue (usually defined as characteristic of wound infection) occur after 48 to 72 hours. Therefore, if an open wound is washed clean every 24 hours, it can be maintained in a nearly sterile condition. This process can be enhanced by the application of a topical antiseptic (not antibiotic) agent. Iodine compounds, mercuric compounds, silver compounds, and other chemicals such as formaldehyde have strong antiseptic properties. Antiseptics kill all types of bacteria, viruses, yeast, and fungi on contact, as opposed to antibiotics, which require metabolism of the toxic agents by bacteria. All of these antiseptics can quickly sterilize a granulating surface. The problem is that most of them injure local tissue or inactivate neutrophils, monocytes, and fibroblasts at the same time. The best antiseptic, and one which renders all others unnecessary, is Dakin's solution and its modifications. Dakin's solution is 0.5% sodium hypochlorite. (Laundry bleach is 5% sodium hypochlorite.) The solution acts by ionization to hypochlorous acid. The hypochlorous acid combines quickly with proteins to produce chloramines, which are toxic to bacteria but not to normal tissues. Tissues tolerate chloramine probably because this is the mechanism of action by which neutrophils kill bacteria, and normal tissues are tolerant of this event. Dakin's solution can be painful on application. This side effect is eliminated by using instead a solution of oxychlorosene (Clorpactin), in which an organic molecule is substituted for the sodium. The release of hypochlorite is even better with this solution than that achieved with Dakin's solution, and bacterial killing is enhanced gram for gram of the active agent.

Based on these principles, the best way to manage an open wound is frequent surgical debridement if necessary, together with extensive local washing followed by loose packing with gauze soaked regularly in oxychlorosene solution. This process is repeated daily. More frequent dressing changes are unnecessary unless the wound is grossly infected or fed by a deeper fistula. These principles apply both to open wounds at the level of the skin and subcutaneous tissue and to deep wounds such as packed open abdominal abscesses, areas of burned skin, and deep open abscesses such as extensive wound infections.

A variation of open wounds are deep infections that have been drained externally but are not amenable to total opening and packing. Examples are pleural space infections, liver abscesses, ischiorectal abscesses, and deep intraperitoneal abscesses. In these conditions, free and open drainage is the primary intent, facilitated by catheter, tube, or suction drainage. Drainage catheters must be large enough to accommodate any particles of debris or granulation tissue in the abscess cavity. The inflammatory margin of granulation tissue (in these examples, the abscess walls) is not accessible for surgical debridement but can and should be soaked with a Dakin's solution equivalent on a regular basis by irrigating through the drainage catheter or through a separate adjacent catheter placed specifically for irrigation.

TABLE 8-2. Host Defense Axioms

1. Massive blood loss is defined as half a blood volume occurring in 24 hours or less. Corollary: surgical intervention is indicated for massive blood loss.
2. The most common cause of postoperative bleeding is "silk-o-penia."
3. Disseminated intravascular coagulation is very rare; localized bleeding with consumption coagulopathy and fibrinolysis is very common.
4. When bleeding persists despite appropriate treatment, this implicates abnormal platelet function. Corollary: there is no good way to measure platelet function. Persistent bleeding after appropriate treatment usually means platelet malfunction.
5. No infusion of platelets or coagulation factors will stop bleeding when the body temperature is less than 35°C.
6. External drainage is always the first treatment of choice for infection. Corollary: antibiotics will not be effective in the treatment of undrained infection.
7. Antiseptics are better than antibiotics for the topical prevention and treatment of surface or body cavity infection.
8. Feed a fever. Full nutrition is the treatment for sepsis.
9. Living on steroids is like living with cancer.
10. Open wounds: Dakin's solution is all you need to know.
11. Wash open wounds, catheter sites, and fresh incisions to prevent infection.

In our case example, we start parenteral and enteral feeding very early. We leave the skin open for 5 days, then perform a delayed primary closure with loose sutures. We use running monofilament polypropylene suture on the fascia to prevent interstices from forming where bacteria could grow; this is supplemented with interrupted heavy absorbable sutures to prevent evisceration in the event of dehiscence. Beginning on the third day, we bathe the patient daily in the tub or shower, taking care to wash thoroughly over the open abdominal wound and around the colostomy, intravenous sites, and bladder catheter. We evacuate stool from the colon proximal and distal to the exteriorized colostomy by using Dakin's solution lavage. We tell the patient to avoid heavy lifting and straining for 6 weeks. We wait 3 months before closing the colostomy.

The important points in host defense physiology and management are summarized in Table 8-2.

Monographs and Reviews

Abraham E. Sepsis: cellular and physiologic mechanisms (New Horizon Series). Baltimore: Williams & Wilkins, Vol. 1, No. 1, 1993.
This multiauthored monograph focuses on research on cytokines and other mediator molecules in the pathophysiology and treatment of systemic sepsis and shock.

Clagett P. Hemostasis in surgical patients. In: Miller TA, Rolands BI, eds. Physiologic basis of modern surgical care. St. Louis: Mosby, 1988.
This is one of the most concise and well-referenced reviews of thrombosis and hemostasis in the modern literature.

Dakin HD, Dunham EK. A handbook of antiseptics. New York: Macmillan, 1918.
The results of Dakin's experiments on topical antiseptics.

Demling R, LaLonde C, Saldinger D, et al. Multiple-organ dysfunction in the surgical patient: pathophysiology, prevention, and treatment. Curr Prob Surg 1993;30:345–410.
An excellent summary of the recent literature.

Fekety R. Antibiotic-associated diarrhea. In: Current Topics in Gastroenterology. New York: Elsevier, 1991.
A thorough review of this problem by one of the first investigators in the field.

Fink MP. Gastrointestinal mucosal injury in experimental models of shock, trauma, and sepsis. Crit Care Med 1991;19:627–40.
This exhaustive literature review describes most of the research related to gut ischemia and its relationship to systemic infection.

Hirsh J. Heparin. N Engl J Med 1991;324:1565–74.

Hirsh J. Oral anticoagulant drugs. N Engl J Med 1991;324:1865–75.
These two reviews summarize the background and modern literature on heparin and oral anticoagulant drugs as well as the current usage protocols.

Jorgensen M, Gustafsen K, Ernst S, Jensen S. Disseminated intravascular coagulation in critically ill patients—laboratory diagnosis. Intensive Care World 1992;9:108–14.

This is a thorough literature review of the laboratory methods used to evaluate coagulation, with an emphasis on the changes that take place during consumption coagulopathy.

Kelly CP, Pothoulakis C, LaMont JT. *Clostridium difficile* colitis. N Engl J Med 1994;330:257-62.

This is a recent review and literature summary on this common ICU problem.

Orgill D, Demling R. Current concepts and approaches to wound healing.. Crit Care Med 1988;16:899-908.

A thorough literature review of the events in wound healing, with emphasis on growth factors and hormones in the enhancement of wound healing.

Rock CS, Lowry SE. Tumor necrosis factor. J Surg Res 1991;51:434-45.

A review of the discovery and study of the most important cytokine identified to date.

Sanford J. Guide to antimicrobial therapy. Dallas: Antimicrobial Therapy, 1993.

This pocket-sized summary of infections and antibiotics prepared by J. Sanford is widely distributed to physicians and medical students by Merck and Company. Because of its wide distribution it has become the standard reference for the use of antimicrobial drugs in intensive care.

Ware JA, Heistad DD. Platelet endothelium interactions. N Engl J Med 1994;328:628-36.

This is a thorough review of the most recent research investigating the adhesion of platelets to endothelium and the formation of the platelet plug.

Weiss SJ. Tissue destruction by neutrophils. N Engl J Med 1989;320:365-76.

This excellent review of neutrophil function as it relates to tissue injury includes a description of the inactivation of oxygen radicals by chloride and protein to form chloramines.

Willmore DW, Smith RJ, O'Dwyer ST, et al. The gut. A central organ after surgical stress. Surgery 1988;104:917-23.

A review of the findings from several studies examining the hypothesis that the intestine is the "motor" of multiple-organ failure. The importance of glutamine in the lumen of the gut is emphasized.

Selected Reports

Baker JW, Deitch EA, Berg RD, Specian RD. Hemorrhagic shock induces bacterial translocation from the gut. J Trauma 1988;28:896-906.

This study demonstrated that bacterial translocation occurs after shock in the rat and the findings indicate that the same phenomenon may take place in patients.

Bernard GR, Loose JM, Sprung CL, et al. Hydrocorticosteroids in patients with the adult respiratory distress syndrome. N Engl J Med 1987;317:1565-70.

This prospective randomized study demonstrated that corticosteroids are not beneficial when given acutely to patients with ARDS. Findings from more recent studies indicate that steroids may be helpful in minimizing fibrosis in late ARDS.

Christou NV, MacLean APH, Meakins JL. Host defense in blunt trauma: interrelationships of kinetics of anergy and depressed neutrophil function, nutritional status, and sepsis. J Trauma 1980;20:833-40.

One of several excellent studies on nutrition and infection, with host defenses measured by skin test reactivity.

Eiseman B, Beart R, Norton L. Multiple organ failure. Surg Gynecol Obstet 1977; 144:323–331.

One of the early clinical papers describing progressive multiple-organ failure.

Gastinne H, Wolff M, Delatour F, et al. A controlled trial in intensive care units of selective decontamination of the digestive tract with nonabsorbable antibiotics. N Engl J Med 1992;326:594–9.

This prospective, randomized double-blind study of 445 patients showed no difference in survival between the group treated with nonabsorbable antibiotics and the group not so treated, and no difference in the incidence of pneumonia, although the diagnosis of pneumonia was not based on culture findings. The study population included patients with a diversity of diagnoses.

Lacroix J, Infante-Rivard C, Jenicek M, Gauthier M. Prophylaxis of upper gastrointestinal bleeding in intensive care units: a meta-analysis. Crit Care Med 1989;17:862–9.

In this review of 15 published studies on this topic the authors concluded that cimetidine and antacids were equally effective in preventing upper gastrointestinal bleeding.

MacLean LD. Delayed type hypersensitivity testing in surgical patients. Surg Gynecol Obstet 1988;166:285–94.

The author summarizes the many contributions of the Montreal group using delayed hypersensitivity as a way of evaluating the metabolism, nutrition, and response to infection. The delayed hypersensitivity test is one of the few practical tests of host defenses that can be used to guide management in critically ill patients.

Michie HR, Manogue KR, Spriggs DR, et al. Detection of circulating tumor necrosis factor after endotoxin administration. N Engl J Med 1988;318:1481–6.

This classic paper describes the physiologic and cytokine effects of endotoxin infusion into normal healthy volunteers.

Pugin J, Aukenthler R, Lew D. Oropharyngeal decontamination decreases incidence of ventilator associated pneumonia. A randomized placebo-control double-blind clinical trial. JAMA 1991;265:2704–10.

A significant decrease in the incidence of nosocomial pneumonia was observed with the oral-gastrointestinal administration of antibiotics. This study has fewer patients but tighter control than the multicenter French study (Gastinne, et al.).

Staab DB, Sorensen VJ, Fath JJ, et al. Coagulation defects resulting from ambient temperature-induced hypothermia. J Trauma 1994;36:634–8.

An excellent study documenting significant coagulopathy resulting from moderate hypothermia.

Van Saene HK, Stoutenbeek CC, Stoller JK. Selective decontamination of the digestive tract in the intensive care unit: current status and future prospects. Crit Care Med 1992;20:691–703.

A meta-analysis of 16 prospective trials of antibiotic-selective decontamination of the gastrointestinal tract. Fifteen of the 16 showed a reduced incidence of infection. The problems associated with blinded randomization are discussed. See the editorial by Fink in this issue of Critical Care Medicine *which points out that, although the incidence of infection is decreased in all of these studies, no beneficial effect on survival has been reported.*

Appendix

I. Basic physics.
   A. Gases.
      1. Boyle's law: At constant *temperature* (T), $P_1V_1 = P_2V_2$.
      2. Charles' law (or Gay-Lussac's law): At constant *pressure* (P), $V_1/V_2 = T_1/T_2$.
      3. Ideal gas law: At constant *volume* (V), P varies directly with T.

         $P_1V_1/T_1 = P_2V_2/T_2$
         or
         $PV = nRT$

         where $R = 0.02$ L/°K and n = moles.

         Using the ideal gas law, the volume of 1 mole at STPD (standard temperature and pressure dry = 0°C [273°K], 760 mm Hg, dry) is 22.4L.
      4. Henry's law: At constant temperature, when a gas and liquid are at equilibrium, the amount of *gas dissolved* in the liquid is directly proportional to the partial pressure of the gas.
      5. Solubility (Bunsen) coefficient at 37°C:

         O_2: 0.023 mL/mL/atm = 0.003 mL/dL/mm Hg
         CO_2: 0.456 mL/mL/atm = 0.006 mL/dL/mm Hg
         N_2: 0.0127 mL/mL/atm = 0.001 mL/dL/mm Hg

B. Hydrodynamics.
  1. Poiseuille's law:

     $$\text{Flow} = P\pi r^4 / 8l\mu$$
     or
     $$\text{Resistance} = 8\mu l / \pi r^4$$

     where P = perfusion pressure gradient; r = vessel radius; 8 = constant; l = length of the vessel; μ = viscosity of the fluid.

     Even though Poiseuille's law applies to the flow of uniform fluids like water through rigid pipes, the principles can be used to understand the factors that control the interrelationships between blood flow and pressure or that govern gas flow through airways related to pressure. The key factor is that flow is directly and linearly related to the pressure gradient and inversely and linearly related to length and viscosity but directly related to the *fourth power* of the radius of the vessel.
  2. Pascal's law: pressure applied to a liquid (or gas) is equally distributed in all directions.
  3. Starling's law of capillary permeability:

     $$Q_f = [K_f(P_v - P_l)] - [\delta(\text{COP} - \text{TOP})]$$

     where Q_f = the net water flow from a capillary bed to the interstitium; $(P_v - P_l)$ = the hydrostatic pressure gradient from the inside to the outside of the capillaries; (COP − TOP) = the pressure gradient created by osmotic pressure inside the capillary (COP) minus the COP in tissue fluid (TOP); K_f = a constant describing the water permeability of the capillary network to water; and δ = the reflectance coefficient, a constant describing the semipermeable nature of the capillary membrane to molecules. Like Poiseuille's law, Starling's law is rarely used for actual calculation but is very helpful for understanding the variables that control the transcapillary filtration of water and small molecules (another way of saying lymph production).

Appendix 215

C. Conversion factors.
1. Temperature:

$$°F = 9/5°C + 32$$
$$°C = 5/9(°F - 32)$$
$$0°C = 273°K$$

2. ATPS (ambient temperature and pressure saturated) to STPD:

$$V_{STPD} = V_{ATPS} \times 273/T + 273 \times P_B - P_{H_2O}/760$$

where P_B = barometric pressure; P_{H_2O} = 47 mm Hg at 37°C; T = °Kelvin.

The factor for converting volume at BTPS (body temperature and pressure saturated, 37°C, 760 mm Hg; P_{H_2O}, 47 mm Hg) is 0.8261. Therefore $V_{STPD} = V_{BTPS} \times 0.8261$.

Factors to Convert Gas Volumes from ATPS to STPD*

Observed P_B (mm Hg)	24°C	26°C	28°C	30°C	32°C
722	0.843	0.833	0.824	0.814	0.804
724	0.845	0.835	0.826	0.816	0.806
726	0.847	0.838	0.829	0.818	0.808
728	0.850	0.840	0.831	0.821	0.811
730	0.852	0.843	0.833	0.823	0.813
732	0.854	0.845	0.836	0.825	0.815
734	0.857	0.847	0.838	0.828	0.818
736	0.859	0.850	0.840	0.830	0.820
738	0.862	0.852	0.843	0.833	0.822
740	0.864	0.855	0.845	0.835	0.825
742	0.867	0.857	0.847	0.837	0.827
744	0.869	0.859	0.850	0.840	0.829
746	0.872	0.862	0.852	0.842	0.832
748	0.874	0.864	0.854	0.845	0.834
750	0.876	0.867	0.857	0.847	0.837
752	0.879	0.869	0.859	0.849	0.839
754	0.881	0.872	0.862	0.852	0.841
756	0.883	0.874	0.864	0.854	0.844
758	0.886	0.876	0.866	0.856	0.846
760	0.888	0.879	0.869	0.859	0.848
762	0.891	0.881	0.871	0.861	0.851
764	0.893	0.884	0.874	0.864	0.853
766	0.896	0.886	0.876	0.866	0.855
768	0.898	0.888	0.878	0.868	0.858
770	0.901	0.891	0.881	0.871	0.860

*Factor $\times V_{ATPS} = V_{STPD}$.

3. Pressure:

   1 mm Hg = 1 torr = 1.36 cm H_2O = 0.133 kPa
   1 Pascal = Pa = 1 newton/m^2
   1 kilopascal = kPa = 1000 N/m^2
   1 kPa = 7.6 mm Hg
   1 newton = N = force that accelerates 1 kg 1 m/s
   1 dyne = force that accelerates 1 g 1 cm/s
   1 atmosphere = 760 mm Hg = 14.7 lbs/sq. in. = 101.3 kPa

4. Temperature correction factors for blood gas measurements: Blood gases are measured at 37°C. At the cooler temperatures more gas is dissolved in water, hence the measured partial pressure will be lower than that measured at 37°C. The opposite is true for temperatures higher than 37°C. The effect of a change in temperature on the partial pressure of CO_2 (P_{CO_2}) and the bicarbonate dissociation curve causes a change in pH, with higher pHs at lower temperatures and vice versa.

5. Basic chemistry conversions:

   1 mole = 1 g molecular weight = 6.023×10^{23} molecules
   1 molar solution = 1 g molecular weight per liter
   1 equivalent = 1 mole divided by valence
   1 g equivalent = weight that will combine with 8.00 g O_2 (1 equivalent of O_2)

Temperature Correction Factors

Patient's Temperature		pH	P_{CO_2}	P_{O_2}
°F	°C		(add to observed values)	
106	41	−0.6	+16%	+25%
105	40.5	−0.5	+14%	+22%
104	40	−0.4	+12%	+19%
103	39.5	−0.4	+10%	+6%
102	39	−0.3	+8%	+13%
101	38.5	−0.2	+6%	+10%
100	38	−0.1	+4%	+7%
98–99	37	None	None	None
97	36	+0.1	−4%	−7%
96	35.5	+0.2	−6%	−10%
95	35	+0.3	−8%	−13%
94	34.5	+0.4	−10%	−16%
93	34	+0.4	−12%	−19%
91	33	+0.6	−16%	−25%
90	32	+0.7	−19%	−30%
88	31	+0.9	−22%	−35%

P_{O_2} = partial pressure of oxygen.

6. Osmolarity:

   a. Osmolality = osmoles/kg of solvent
      Osmolarity = osmoles/liter of solvent
      1 mole/liter depresses freezing point of water 1.86°C
      Number of mOsm/L = Δ freezing point/0.00186
      1 osmole = molecular weight/particles/molecule
      1 Osm/L = 1000 mOsm/L
      1 Osm NaCl = 58.5 g/2 = 29.25 g of NaCl = 1000 mOsm/L
      Normal toxicity = 300 mOsm/L = 0.9 g/dL of NaCl

   A quick bedside estimate of osmolality is:

   Plasma osmolality = [2 × (Na + K)] + [BUN/2.8] + [glucose/18]

   b. Osmotic pressure (same as ideal gas law):

      $P = nRT/V$

      where P = pressure in mm Hg; n = moles; R = 0.02 L/°K, T = °K; V = volume.
      Colloid osmotic pressure: Pressure generated by small charged molecules electrically obligated to remain close to large charged protein molecules.

7. Standard international units: In the Système International, concentration is expressed as moles (or nano-, micro-, or millimoles) per liter. Despite the efforts of many editors, it has not been adopted in the United States. (Campion E. A retreat from SI units. N Engl J Med 1992;327:49.)

II. Body surface area.

Dubois formula: BSA = $W^{0.0425} \times H^{0.725} \times 71.84$

where BSA = body surface area; W = weight; and H = height.
A nomogram based on this equation is shown in Figure A-1.

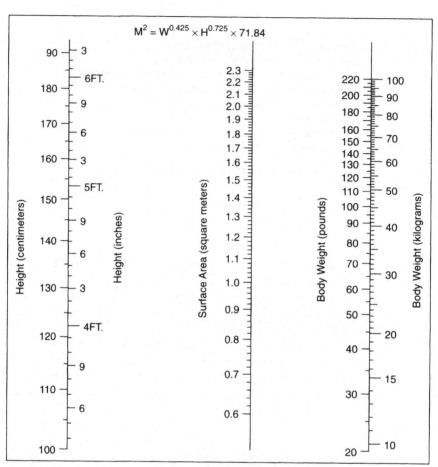

FIGURE A-1. Surface area calculated from height (*H*) and weight (*W*). Nomogram constructed from the Du Bois–Meeh formula for surface area.

III. Equations
   A. Alveolar air equation:

   $$P_{AO_2} = ([F_{iO_2}(713)] - P_{aCO_2})(F_{iO_2} + 1 - F_{iO_2}/RQ)$$

   The alveolar air equation is used to calculate the percentage of oxygen (or the PO_2) in end-tidal alveolar gas, when the inspired oxygen concentration (F_{iO_2}) and the arterial P_{aCO_2} ($[P_{aCO_2}]$ or end-tidal P_{CO_2}) are known. A simplifed version of the alveolar air equation used for most clinical circumstances. is:

   $$P_{AO_2} = P_{iO_2} - P_{ACO_2}$$

   where P_{AO_2} = end-tidal alveolar P_{O_2}; $P_{iO_2} = F_{iO_2}(P_B - P_{H_2O})$; and $P_{ACO_2} = P_{aCO_2}$ or end-tidal P_{CO_2} if lung function is nearly normal. P_{H_2O} at 37°C is 47 mm Hg, so that at normal P_B at sea level $P_B - P_{H_2O} = 760 - 47 = 713$.

   If the volume of oxygen absorbed ($\dot{V}_{O_2}$) is exactly the same as the volume of CO_2 excreted ($\dot{V}_{CO_2}$) ($\dot{V}_{CO_2}/\dot{V}_{O_2}$ is 1.0; respiratory quotient [RQ] = 1.0), then the alveolar air equation is correct as just stated. However, if the RQ is more or less than 1, then the P_{ACO_2} part of the equation must be corrected to account for this small volume change. The correction factor is $F_{iO_2} + 1 - F_{iO_2}$ divided by RQ. If the RQ is 0.8 (as is commonly assumed), the correction factor is 1.2. When the P_{ACO_2} is multiplied by 1.2, the final calculation of P_{AO_2} is affected by a few millimeters mercury.

   The derivation of this correction factor is based on the fact that the amount of nitrogen gas in inhaled and exhaled air is exactly the same, although the concentration of nitrogen in exhaled gas might be slightly higher in exhaled gas, therefore:

   $$\dot{V} \text{ inspired } (1 - F_{iO_2} - F_{iCO_2}) = \dot{V} \text{ expired } (1 - F_{AO_2} - F_{ACO_2})$$

   where $\dot{V}$ = volume; F_{iCO_2} = fraction of inspired CO_2; F_{AO_2} = fraction of oxygen in alveolar gas; F_{ACO_2} = fraction of CO_2 in alveolar gas.

   When actual values for $\dot{V}_{O_2}$ and $\dot{V}_{CO_2}$ are substituted into this equation, the correction factor results.

   For clinical purposes, and even for most clinical physiologic studies, the P_B is assumed to be 760 mm Hg, the temperature is assumed to be 37°C (hence the P_{H_2O} of 47 mm Hg), and the RQ is assumed to be 1.0. At actual elevations up to 1,000 feet (300 meters) above sea level, P_B typically ranges from 740 to 770 mm Hg. The patient's temperature, or the temperature of the exhaled gas in which end-tidal CO_2 is measured, might range from 30° to 40°C. The RQ in most ICU patients who are being provided with appropriate nutrition should be 1.0; however, it may range from 0.6 in a starving patient to 1.3 in a patient who is being fed an excess amount of carbohydrate. Another potential source of error is that the F_ICO_2 is not zero, as is assumed in the alveolar air equation, but is some fraction slightly greater than zero, representing the amount of CO_2 in the conducting airways at the time the patient initiated an inspiratory breath. An additional potential source of error is the F_IO_2, which is rarely measured to two decimal places, which would be required for absolute accuracy. Even if all of these respiratory parameters for which there is a potential error in their measurement were measured precisely and calculated appropriately, the effect on the calculated P_AO_2 would be small (perhaps 5 to 10 mm Hg). Therefore the simplified version of the alveolar air equation, without all the technically proper correction factors, is used most of the time. Altitude is corrected for if the location is more than 1000 feet (300 meters) above sea level. Although many textbooks advocate using a correction factor for the RQ assuming that RQ is 0.8, this assumption is no more accurate than assuming that the RQ is 1.0.

B. Pulmonary shunt.

The formula for calculating the transpulmonary shunt is:

$$\dot{Q}s/\dot{Q}t = \frac{CcO_2 - CaO_2}{CcO_2 - CvO_2}$$

where $\dot{Q}s$ = blood flowing through the lung without participating in gas exchange; $\dot{Q}t$ = cardiac output; CcO_2 = content of blood leaving pulmonary capillaries after equilibrating with alveolar air; CaO_2 = arterial oxygen content; and CvO_2 = venous oxygen content.

The derivation of the shunt equation is as follows: The Fick axiom is that $\dot{V}O_2$ across the functioning pulmonary capillaries is equal to the amount of oxygen consumed in peripheral tissue metabolism; therefore using the Fick equation:

$$Qp = \dot{V}O_2/(CcO_2 - CvO_2)$$

where $\dot{Q}p$ = blood flowing through ideally functioning pulmonary capillaries in which the content of exiting blood is equilibrated with alveolar gas. The oxygen content of this idealized pulmonary venous blood, designated CcO_2, is calculated as the hemoglobin concentration (in grams per deciliter) × 1.36 × percent saturation + P_AO_2 × 0.003 cc/dL/mm Hg. The idealized saturation is always 100% if the subject is breathing more than 20% oxygen; 1.36 is the oxygen binding capacity per gram of hemoglobin; P_AO_2 is the P_O_2 in alveolar gas derived from the alveolar air equation; and 0.003 is the solubility coefficient for oxygen at 37°C.

Also using the Fick equation:

$$\dot{Q}t = \dot{V}O_2/(CaO_2 - CvO_2)$$

where $\dot{Q}t$ = total blood flow through the systemic or pulmonary circulation (that is, the cardiac output).

The amount of blood flowing through the pulmonary circulation, but not through functional capillaries (the transpulmonary shunt), is therefore $\dot{Q}t - \dot{Q}p$.

Therefore the ratio of the shunt flow to the total flow is

$$\dot{Q}s/\dot{Q}t = \dot{Q}t - (\dot{Q}p/\dot{Q}t)$$

Substituting the definitions for $\dot{Q}p$ and $\dot{Q}t$:

$$\dot{Q}s/\dot{Q}t = \frac{\dot{V}O_2/(CaO_2 - CvO_2) - \dot{V}O_2/(CcO_2 - CvO_2)}{\dot{V}O_2/(CaO_2 - CvO_2)},$$

This equation simplified becomes:

$$\dot{Q}s/\dot{Q}t = (CcO_2 - CaO_2)/(CcO_2 - CvO_2)$$

It is worth noting that, in Julius Comroe's classic textbook on the lung, the shunt equation is derived in a different fashion and the final result is $(CaO_2 - CcO_2)/(CvO_2 - CcO_2)$, so that the calculation is always done with negative values but the final ratio is the same as that calculated using the classic derivation just shown.

C. Respiratory dead space.

The formula for calculating the respiratory dead space ($\dot{V}D$) is:

$$\dot{V}D = [(F_ACO_2 - F_ECO_2)\dot{V}E]/F_ACO_2$$

where F_ACO_2 = fraction of CO_2 in alveolar gas; and F_ECO_2 = fraction of CO_2 in mixed expired gas.

The derivation of this equation is as follows:

$$\dot{V}E = \dot{V}A + \dot{V}D$$

where $\dot{V}E$ = the volume of exhaled gas; $\dot{V}A$ = the volume of gas that came from alveoli; and $\dot{V}D$ = the volume of gas that came from dead space. Dead space here is considered to be the conducting airways plus any alveolar space that is ventilated without any gas exchange. The amount of gas (G) in these volumes is:

$$F_{E_G} \times \dot{V}E(F_{A_G} \times \dot{V}A) + (F_{D_G} \times \dot{V}D)$$

where F_{E_G} = fraction of gas (G) in mixed expired gas; F_{A_G} = fraction of gas (G) in alveolar gas; and F_{D_G} = fraction of gas (G) in dead space gas.

The concentration of any gas in the dead space is:

$$F_{D_G} = F_{I_G}$$

where F_{I_G} = fraction of gas (G) in inspired gas.

Therefore:

$$F_{E_G} \times \dot{V}E = (F_{A_G} \times \dot{V}A) + (F_{I_G} \times \dot{V}D)$$

Therefore:

$$F_{E_G} \times \dot{V}_E = [F_{A_G}(\dot{V}_E - \dot{V}_D)] + F_{I_G}\dot{V}_D$$

and

$$\dot{V}_D = [(F_{A_G} - F_{E_G}) \times \dot{V}_E]/F_{A_G} - F_{I_G}$$

When the gas is carbon dioxide, $F_{I_G} = 0$ and the final equation becomes:

$$\dot{V}_D = [(F_ACO_2 - F_ECO_2) \times \dot{V}_E]/F_ACO_2$$

The concentration of CO_2 in alveolar gas is assumed to be the same as that in arterial blood. Therefore the equation can be restated as:

$$\dot{V}_D/\dot{V}_E = (PaCO_2 - P_ECO_2)/PaCO_2$$

Mixed expired P_{CO_2} is typically 26 mm Hg at STPD; therefore in a normal person:

$$\dot{V}_D = (40 - 26)/40 = 34\%$$

D. Harris-Benedict equation for determining basal metabolic rate.

Men: EE = 66.5 + 13.7W + 5.00H − 6.78A
Women: EE = 65.5 + 9.56W + 1.85H − 4.68A

where EE = energy expenditure; W = weight; H = height; and A = age.

(Benedict FG. A study of prolonged fasting. Washington, DC: Carnegie Institute, 1915, Pub. No. 203.)

E. Equation for indirect calorimetry.

The simple equation for indirect calorimetry assumes that the RQ is 1.0 and the caloric value of all substrates consumed in metabolism is 5 kcal/L of oxygen consumed; therefore the simple equation for indirect calorimetry is:

$\dot{V}_{O_2}$ in L/min × 60 min/hr × 24 hr/day × 5 kcal/L O_2 = kcal/day

or

$\dot{V}_{O_2}$ in L/min × 7.2 = kcal/day

This equation oversimplifies several factors. The oxygen consumption value of carbohydrate is 5 cal/L of oxygen but the $\dot{V}_{O_2}$ for protein is 4.8 cal/L of oxygen and that for fat is 4.7 cal/L of oxygen. Furthermore, the RQ for carbohydrate is 1, for protein 0.8, and for fat 0.7. The amount of protein substrate that is metabolized can be calculated from the amount of nitrogen in urine during a timed collection. For example, if a 24-hour urine sample contains 10 g of nitrogen, then 62.5 g of protein was metabolized to produce this amount of nitrogen (most of it as urea). The metabolism of 62.5 g of protein would consume 52 L of oxygen and produce 42 L of CO_2. If the total amount of oxygen consumed and CO_2 produced is measured, then the amount accounted for by protein metabolism can be subtracted and the amount resulting from carbohydrate and fat metabolism can be calculated from these corrected values. Therefore the exact amount of protein, fat, and carbohydrate that went to make up the overall metabolism can be calculated and the exact values for conversion of the $\dot{V}_{O_2}$ to calories can be calculated. All of these variables are included in the Weir equation as follows:

cal/day = [(3.941 × $\dot{V}_{O_2}$) + (1.106 × $\dot{V}_{CO_2}$)] − (2.17 × g urinary N/day)

(Weir JB ed: New methods for calculating metabolic rate with special reference to protein metabolism. J Physiol 1949:109:1–9.)

F. The Sargent equation for the calculation of the protein catabolic rate. Patients in renal failure do not maintain a stable blood urea nitrogen (BUN) level, but the change in the BUN concentration during a period can be used to calculate the amount of protein metabolized to produce that amount of urea nitrogen. The concentration of urea must be corrected for the fact that urea is diluted in total body water, so that an estimate of change in extracellular fluid must be taken into account when making this calculation. The Sargent formula, taking all these variables into account, is as follows:

Protein catabolic rate = $(N_{excreted} + N_{accumulated}) \times 6.25$

where $N_{excreted}$ = urea N excreted (typically 8–10 g/day) plus non–urea N (typically 1.5 g/d); and $N_{accumulated} = BUN_2 \times TBW_2 - BUN_1 \times TBW_1$, where BUN_2 = urea N in g/dL at time 2; TBW_2 = total body water in dL at time 2; BUN_2, TBW_2 = same at time 1; and TBW = best estimate of TBW (lean, dry = 58% weight; obese = 40% weight).

Fluid overloaded = 58% dry weight + kg over dry weight and 6.25 g of protein = g of N.

(Sargent J, Gotch F, Borah M, et al. Urea kinetics: a guide to nutritional management of acute renal failure. Am J Clin Nutr 1978;31:1696–702.

G. Henderson-Hasselbalch equation. This equation is basically the equilibration equation for the carbonic acid–bicarbonate buffer system. The equation is:

$$pH = pKa + \log \frac{[A^-]}{[HA]} = 6.1 \log \frac{[HCO_3^-]}{[CO_2]}$$

where [HA] = the concentration of the free acid; [A$^-$] = the concentration of the ionized form; and pKa = the negative logarithm of the dissociation constant (K_a); hence [CO_2] = the sum of the dissolved CO_2 and HCO_3^-.

(Henderson LJ. A critical study of the process of acid excretion. J Biol Chem 1911;9:403–24.)

IV. Scoring systems.
   A. Trauma Scores.
      1. Acute injury score (AIS-85).

         Score: head/neck, 0–5; face, 0–5; thorax, 0–5; abdomen, 0–5; extremities, 0–5; external, 0–5.
         Range: 0 = normal; 1 = minimal, 2 = moderate; 3 = severe, not life-threatening; 4 = severe, life-threatening; 5 = critical, survival uncertain.
         LD50: Convert to injury severity score (ISS).
         (The Abbreviated Injury Scale (AIS)—1985 revision. Des Plaines, IL: American Association of Automotive Medicine; Civil I, Schwab W. The abbreviated injury scale, 1985 revision. A condensed chart for clinical use. J Trauma 1988;28:87–90.)
      2. Injury severity score (ISS, Baker).

         Score: square AIS for each region, then sum.
         Range: 0 (normal) to 75 (arbitrary maximum).
         LD50: 35.
         Example:

	AIS	AIS Squared
Mild closed head injury	3 →	9
Ruptured spleen	4 →	16
Fractured femur	3 →	9
ISS		34

         (Baker SP, O'Neill B, Haddon W, et al. The injury severity score: a method for describing patients with multiple injury and evaluating emergency care. J Trauma 1974;14:187–96.)
      3. Trauma score (Champion).

Respiratory Rate	Respiratory Effort	Blood Pressure	Capillary Refill	Glasgow Coma Score
0–4	0–1	0–4	0–2	1–5

         Score: 0 = critical; high = normal.
         Range: 16 (normal) to 1.
         LD50: 10.
         (Champion HR, Sacco WJ, Hunt TK. Trauma severity scoring to predict mortality. World J Surg 1983;7:4–11.)
      4. TRISS (Boyd). The TRISS (*trauma/i*njury *s*everity *s*core) is a mortality prediction score based on the ISS and patient's age, an admission physiology score, and the type of injury. LD50 = 50 points.
         (Boyd CR, Tolson MA, Copes WS. Evaluating trauma care: the TRISS method. J Trauma 1987;27:370.)

5. 24-hour ICU point system (Sacramento).

Variable	Points
Glasgow Coma Scale Score	
13–15	0
9–12	1
6–8	2
4–5	3
3	4
PaO$_2$/FiO$_2$	
>325	0
225–324	1
175–224	2
125–174	3
<125	4
Fluid balance (liters)	
<3	0
>3	4

Sum points = score.
LD50 = 7.5 points.
(Vassar M, Wilkerson BH, Duran PJ, et al. Comparison of APACHE II, TRISS, and a proposed 24-hour point system for predicting outcome in ICU trauma patients. J Trauma 1992;32:490–500.)

B. Acute physiology scores.
  1. APACHE. There are three versions of the *a*cute *p*hysiology *a*nd chronic *h*ealth *e*valuation described by Knaus. Only APACHE II and APACHE III are now in use. APACHE II is described here and is intended as an ICU admission, one-time scoring system. APACHE III is based on similar information that is collected and analyzed daily and reported as the mortality risk on that day compared with the thousands of patients in the central registry. APACHE III requires a computer program and participation in the central registry.
  The APACHE II Score: acute physiology score plus age factor plus past history factor.
  Range: 0 (normal) to 56.
  LD50: 20–25.
  (Knaus WA, Draper EA, Wagner DP, et al. APACHE II: A severity of disease classification system. Crit Care Med 1985;13:818–29.)
  2. Concomitant organ failure (NIH—ECMO study, 1975–78)

No. of organs	Mortality risk
Respiratory only	40%
Two-organ failure	55%
Three-organ failure	75%
Four-organ failure	85%
Five-organ failure	100%

(Bartlett RH, Morris AH, Fairley HB, et al. A prospective study of acute hypoxic respiratory failure. Chest 1986;89:684–9.)

3. Specific organ failure (single or multiple) (UMSICU, 1991).

	Mortality
Respiratory	22%
Renal	38%
Liver	27%
Cardiac	67%
Infection	28%

(Bartlett RH: Critical Care Handbook, Ann Arbor: Department of Surgery, University of Michigan, 1993.)

4. Systemic inflammatory responses/sepsis (SIRS) definitions.
   SIRS 2 or more:
   a. Temperature: $>38°C$ or $<36°C$
   b. Pulse: >90 beats/min
   c. Respiration: >20 breaths/min
   d. White blood cell count: $>12/mm^3$ or $<4,000/mm^3$

   Sepsis: SIRS plus positive culture results.
   Severe sepsis: Sepsis with organ dysfunction.
   Septic shock: Sepsis with hypotension despite treatment.
   Culture-negative sepsis: Definitions as above with patient on antibiotics but with negative culture findings.

5. Organ dysfunction:
   a. Respiratory: PaO_2/FiO_2, <175; positive chest x-ray findings; pulmonary capillary wedge pressure, <18 mm Hg.
   b. Renal: creatinine, >20 mg/dL
   c. Coagulopathy: platelet count, 25%, increased prothrombin time.
   d. Central nervous system: Glasgow coma score.

(American College of Chest Physician's Society of Critical Care Medicine Consensus Conference: Definitions for sepsis and organ failure and guidelines for use of innovative therapies in sepsis. Crit Care Med 1992;20:864–75.)

6. SIRS/sepsis score.

Status	Mortality	"Culture Negative"
SIRS	12%	NA
Sepsis	16%	10%
Severe sepsis	20%	10%
Septic shock	46%	46%

(Rangel-Fransto M, Pittet D, Costigan M, et al. The natural history of the systemic inflammatory response syndrome [SIRS]: a prospective study. JAMA 1995;273: 117–123; ACCP-SCCM: Definitions for sepsis and organ failure and guidelines for the use of innovative therapies in sepsis. Crit Care Med 1992;26:864.)

The APACHE II Severity of Disease Classification System

Physiologic Variable	High Abnormal Range				Normal	Low Abnormal Range		
	+4	+3	+2	+1	0	+1	+2	+3
Temperature, rectal (°C)	≥41°	39°–40.9°	—	38.5°–38.9°	36°–38.4°	34°–35.9°	32°–33.9°	30°–31.9°
Mean arterial pressure (mm Hg)	≥160	130–159	110–129	—	70–109	—	50–69	—
Heart rate (ventricular response) (beats/min)	≥180	140–179	110–139	—	70–109	—	55–69	40–54
Respiratory rate (nonventilated or ventilated) (breaths/min)	≥50	35–49	—	25–34	12–24	10–11	6–9	—
Oxygenation: $AaDO_2$ or PaO_2 (mm Hg)								
a. $FiO_2 \geq 0.5$; record $AaDO_2$	≥500	350–499	200–349	—	<200	—	—	—
b. $FiO_2 < 0.5$; record only PaO_2	—	—	—	—	$PO_2 > 70$	PO_2 61–70	—	PO_2 55–60
Arterial pH	≥7.7	7.6–7.69	—	7.5–7.59	7.33–7.49	—	7.25–7.32	7.15–7.24
Serum sodium (mmol/L)	≥180	160–179	155–159	150–154	130–149	—	120–129	111–119
Serum potassium (mmol/L)	≥7	6–6.9	—	5.5–5.9	3.5–5.4	3–3.4	2.5–2.9	—
Serum creatinine (mg/dL) (double-point score for acute renal failure)	≥3.5	2–3.4	1.5–1.9	—	0.6–1.4	—	<0.6	—
Hematocrit (%)	≥60	—	50–59.9	46–49.9	30–45.9	—	20–29.9	—
White blood cell count (Total/mm³) (in 1,000s)	≥40	—	20–39.9	15–19.9	3–14.9	—	1–2.9	—
GCS score = 15—actual GCS score.								
A Total APS. Sum of the 12 individual variable points.								
Serum HCO_3^- (venous—mmol/L) (Not preferred; use if no ABGs)	≥52	41–51.9	—	32–40.9	22–31.9	—	18–21.9	15–17.9

B Age points

Assign points to age as follows:

Age (yrs)	Points
≤44	0
45–54	2
55–64	3
66–74	5
≥75	6

C Chronic health points:

If the patient has a history of severe organ system insufficiency or is immunocompromised, assign points as follows:

a. For nonoperative or emergency postoperative patients—5 points, or

b. For elective postoperative patients—2 points.

Definitions:

Organ insufficiency or immunocompromised state must have been evident **prior** to this hospital admission and conform to the following criteria:

Liver: Biopsy-proven cirrhosis and documented portal hypertension; episodes of past upper GI tract bleeding attributed to portal hypertension; or prior episodes of hepatic failure/encephalopathy/coma.

Cardiovascular: New York Heart Association functional class IV.

Respiratory: Chronic restrictive, obstructive, or vascular disease resulting in severe exercise restriction, e.g., unable to climb stairs or perform household duties; or documented chronic hypoxia, hypercapnia, secondary polycythemia, severe pulmonary hypertension (>40 mm Hg), or respirator dependency.

Renal: Receiving chronic dialysis. Immunocompromised: the patient has received therapy that suppresses resistance to infection, e.g., immunosuppression treatment, chemotherapy/radiation, long-term or recent high-dose steroid therapy; or has a disease that is sufficiently advanced to suppress resistance to infection, e.g., leukemia, lymphoma, AIDS.

APACHE II SCORE

Sum of A + B

A APS points _____
B Age points _____
C Chronic health points _____
Total APACHE II _____

$AaDO_2$ = alveolar-arterial gradient for oxygen; ABGs = arterial blood gases; APS = acute physiology score; FiO_2 = fraction of inspired oxygen; GCS = Glasgow coma score; PaO_2 = arterial oxygen pressure; Po_2 = partial pressure of oxygen.

C. Adult respiratory distress syndrome (ARDS) scoring systems.
   1. Murray lung score (1988).

X-ray Study	PaO_2/FiO_2	Compliance	PEEP (cm H_2O)	Score	Approximate Mortality
Normal	>300	>1.0	<5	0	0
One quadrant	255–299	0.4–0.9	6–8	1	25%
Two quadrants	175–224	0.4–0.7	9–11	2	50%
Three quadrants	100–174	0.2–0.4	12–14	3	75%
Four quadrants	<100	<0.2	>15	4	90%

PEEP = positive end-expiratory pressure.
(Murray JF, Matthay MA, Luce LM, et al. An expanded definition of the adult respiratory distress syndrome. Am Rev Respir Dis 1988;138:720–3.)

   2. Geneva score (Morel, 1985).

X-ray Study	$AaDO_2/FiO_2$	Compliance	EIP (cm H_2O)	Score	Approximate Mortality
Normal	<300	>1.0	<20	0	0
Interstitial	300–375	0.6–0.9	20–25	1	25%
Interstitial	375–450	0.5–0.7	25–30	2	50%
Consolidation	450–525	0.3–0.5	30–35	3	75%
Consolidation	>525	<0.3	>35	4	90%

EIP = end inspiratory pressure.
(Morel D, Dargent F, Bachman M, et al. Pulmonary extraction of serotonin and propranolol in patients with ARDS. Am Rev Respir Dis 1985;132:475–84.)

   3. Euroxy Study (Artigas, 1991).

X-ray Study	PaO_2 (mm Hg)	FiO_2	PEEP (cm H_2O)	Tidal Volume (cc/kg)	Score	Approximate Mortality
Infiltrate	>75	0.5	5	10	Hypoxic	38%
Infiltrate	<75	0.5	5	10	Severe	69%

(Artigas A, Carlet J, McGall JR, et al. Clinical presentation prognostic factors and outcome of ARDS in the European collaborative study [1985–1987]. In: Zapol W, Lemare F, eds. Adult respiratory distress syndrome. New York: Dekker, 1991:37–63.)

   4. Massachusetts General Hospital score (Zapol, 1991).

X-ray study	Ventilation	Oxygen	Severity	Mortality
Minimal	+/− Intubate	$FiO_2 < 0.5$	Mild	18%
Panlobular	PPV	$FiO_2 > 0.5$	Moderate	49%
Bilateral	PPV + PEEP	$FiO_2 > 0.6$ or $PaO_2 < 50$ mm Hg	Severe	84%

PPV = positive-pressure ventilation.
(Zapol WM, Frikker MJ, Pontoppidian H, et al. The adult respiratory distress syndrome at Massachusetts General Hospital. In: Zapol W, Lemare F, eds. Adult Respiratory Distress Syndrome. New York: Dekker, 1991:367–80.)

Appendix

D. Liver Failure (Child, 1960).

Class	Bilirubin (mg/dL)	Albumin (g/dL)	Ascites	Encephalopathy	Malnutrition
A	<2	>3.5	0	0	0
B	2–3	3–3.5	Mild	Mild	Mild
C	>3	<3	Severe	Severe	Severe

(Child CG. Hepatic circulation and portal hypertension. Philadelphia: Saunders, 1954.)

E. Pancreatitis (Ranson, 1974).

Admission Findings	48-Hour Findings
Age, >55 yr	Hematocrit ↑ 10%
Glucose, >200 mg/dL	BUN ↑ 5 mg/dL
LDH, >300 Iu/L	Calcium <8 mg/dL
SGOT, >250 IU	PaO_2 <60 mm Hg
WBC, >16,000/mm^3	BBD >4 mEq/L
	Fluid >6 L

BBD = buffer base deficit; LDH = lactate dehydrogenase; SGOT = transaminase.

Positive Signs	Mortality
3–4	15%
5–6	50%
7+	80%+

(Ransom JAC, Rivkind KM, et al. Prognostic signs and role of operative management in acute pancreatitis. Surg Gynecol Obstet 1974;139:69.)

F. Cardiac system abnormalities.
  1. Myocardial infarction (Killip, 1967).

NYHA Class	Cardiac Failure	Ejection Fraction	Mortality (1967)
I	None	0.47	8%
II	Mild	0.36	30%
III	Pulmonary edema	0.31	44%
IV	Cardiogenic shock	0.12	80%+

NYHA = New York Heart Association.
(Killip T, Kimball JT. Treatment of myocardial infarction in a coronary care unit. A two-year experience with 250 patients. Am J Cardiol 1967;20:457.)

  2. Cardiogenic shock (Balakumaran, 1986).

Hemodynamic Parameters	NYHA Class			
	I	II	III	IV
Heart rate (beats/min)	70–85	85–100	90–110	>110
Systolic BP mm Hg	>90	80–90	60–80	<60
PCWP (mm Hg)	<12	12–14	14–18	>18
CI	>3	2.5–3	2–2.5	<2
LVSWI	>270	200–270	120–200	<120
Approximate mortality	10%	25%	40%	60%

BP = blood pressure; CI = cardiac index; LVSWI = left ventricular stroke work index; PCWP = pulmonary capillary wedge pressure.
(Balakumaran K, Hugenholz P. Cardiogenic shock; current concepts in management. Drugs 1986;32:372.)

Index

Abscesses, 196
Acid-base physiology, 165–173
Acidosis, 168, 169, 170, 172–173
Acquired immune deficiency syndrome (AIDS), 198, 203
Activated clotting time (ACT), 188, 189
Acute injury score, 225
Acute physiology scores, 226–229
Acute renal failure (ARF), 115–116, 136–143
  algorithm, 140
  axioms, 152
  drug-induced, 138
  pharmacology, 151–152
  prognosis, 150–151
Acute tubular necrosis (ATN), 136, 137
Adult respiratory distress syndrome (ARDS), 70, 72–73, 93, 201
  scoring systems, 230
Advanced Cardiac Life Support Manual, 41–42
AIDS. *See* Acquired immune deficiency syndrome
Alkalosis, 168, 169, 170, 172, 173
Alveolar air equation, 219–220
Alveolar collapse, 65–68
Anemia, 11, 12, 25, 28
Anion gap, 172
Antibiotics, 199, 200
APACHE score system, 226, 228–229

Arrhythmia, 43–45
Arterial oxygen content. *See* Oxygen content, arterial blood
Arteriovenous oxygen content difference ($AVDO_2$), 3, 4, 6, 10, 11, 17, 18
  cardiac output, 34–35
Assist-control ventilation, 80, 90
Assisted ventilation, 80
Autoregulation
  blood flow, 35, 66, 178–180
  filling pressure, 27–29
  to maintain oxygen delivery, 11

Bacterial infections, 194–197, 199, 202–203
Balanced-salt solution, 162
Base deficit, 167–168
Base excess, 168, 171, 172
Bicarbonate buffer system, 168, 169–171
Bleeding, 183, 184–187
  abnormalities, 190–193
  algorithm, 193
Blood
  carbon dioxide content, 63
  clotting, 184–185, 186, 187, 190–193
  oxygen content. *See* Oxygen content
  volume, 24–45, 155–156

Blood flow, 35–36, 178–180
Blood pressure, 25
  measurement, 30–32
  normal value, 30
Body composition, 155–157
Body surface area, 217–218
Breathing, 48, 55–61

Caloric expenditure of metabolism, 5, 10, 105
Calorimetry, indirect, 102–103, 223
Carbohydrates, 103–104, 106
  in feeding formulas, 119, 124
  stored, 109
Carbon dioxide
  kinetics, 61–65
  measurement of, 62–63
  transfer in the lung, 63–65
Cardiac function, 24–29, 231
Cardiac index, 3, 5, 9, 10, 36
  normal value, 30
Cardiac output, 2, 5, 13, 15
  autoregulation, 25
  measurement, 32–35
  normal value, 30
  during respiratory failure, 76
Cardiogenic shock, scoring system, 231
Catecholamine secretion, 11, 25
Catheters
  blood pressure monitoring, 30–31, 36
  fiberoptic-equipped, 8
  infection from, 125, 197, 202
  renal replacement therapy, 145–146, 147
Central blood volume, 32
Central venous pressure, 26, 29
  normal value, 30
Cerebral blood flow, 178–180
Cholestasis, 120, 122
Clark electrode, 6–7
Closed-circuit rebreathing volumetric spirometry, 2–3
Clots
  blood, 185, 186, 187, 189, 190–193
  cryoprecipitate, 192
Coagulopathy, 190–193

Collagen, 184, 186, 196, 204–205
Coma, 176–178
Consciousness, 176–178
Continuous arteriovenous hemofiltration (CAVH), 144, 146–147, 148
Continuous hemodiafiltration, 148–149
Continuous venovenous hemfiltration (CVVH), 147
Controlled mechanical ventilation (CMV), 80, 90
Conversion factors, 215–216
Creatinine, 111, 152
Cryoprecipitate, 192
Cushing's ulcer, 123

Dakin's solution, 207, 208
DC fibrillator, 44
Dextrose, 162, 164
Dialysate solution, 148–149
Diarrhea, during enteral feeding, 119, 120
Drug dosages
  during acute renal failure, 151
  antibiotics, 200

Edema, 28, 92–95, 194
Effective compliance, 52
Electrocardiography, 41–43
Electroencephalography, 180
Electrolyte balance
  during acute renal failure, 139
  during starvation, 164–165
  and water, 159–161
Electrolytes, 155–173
  algorithm, 166
  axioms, 173
  replacement of, 162–164
Energy balance, 113–117
  during acute renal failure, 141
  vs. nitrogen balance, 118
Energy reserves, 111
Energy sources, 103–106, 109–113
Enteral feeding, 117, 119–123
  formulas, 121
  guidelines, 127
Equations, 219–224

Erythropoietin, 11
Euglobulin lysis time, 189
Euroxy Study, 230
Exercise, 11, 13–15, 19
Extracellular fluids, 155, 156–157, 159
Extracorporeal membrane oxygenation (ECMO), 77

Factor XII, 185, 188, 190, 192
Fasting, metabolism during, 109–110, 164
Fats, 104, 106
  body composition, 156
  catabolism of, 110
  in feeding formulas, 121, 124–125
  stored energy reserves, 109, 111
Fibrin, 184–185, 186, 187
  formation, 188–189, 204
Fibrin degradation products (FDPs), 189, 190, 191
Fibrinogen, 191
Fibrinolysis, 189, 190
Fibrosis, 183, 204–205
Fick equation, 2, 3, 18, 30
Fick method, 34–35
Flow cytometry, 198
Fluids, 155–173
  algorithm, 166
  axioms, 173
  and electrolyte replacement, 162–164
  exchanges with environment, 157–158
  pathologic losses, 157
  patient management, 164–165
  third-space loss, 156, 157–158
Formulas (feeding)
  enteral, 119–120, 121
  parenteral, 124, 126
Frank-Starling curve, 26, 27, 93
Function residual capacity (FRC), 25, 31, 53–54
  during alveolar collapse, 65–66
  during mechanical ventilation, 89

Gases, 55–61, 213
Gastrointestinal tract bleeding, 122–123
Geneva score, 230

Glascow coma scale, 176–178
Glucose, administration, 103
Granulation tissue, 194, 196, 206

Hageman factor. *See* Factor XII
Harris-Benedict equation, 222
Hartman's solution, 162
Head trauma, 181
Healing, tissue, 183, 204–205
Hemodialysis, 143–145
Hemodynamics, 24–45
  axioms, 41
  normal values, 30
  of shock, 37–38
Hemoglobin, oxygen content, 5–6, 7–8
Henderson-Hasselbalch equation, 167, 168–171, 224
Homeostasis. *See* Autoregulation
Host defense mechanisms, 183–209
  axioms, 208–209
Hydrodynamics, physics of, 214
Hyperdynamic response, 18, 40–41
Hyperglycemia, 125
Hyperkalemia, 139, 141
Hypertension, drugs used, 40
Hypervolemia, 28, 29
Hypoperfusion, 36–41
Hypoproteinemia, 28, 127
Hypotension, 28, 36–41
Hypothermia, 18
Hypovolemia, 25, 28, 29, 36, 138, 164
Hypoxia, 11, 12, 25

Immunosuppression, 198, 203, 206
Indicator dilution method, 32–34
Indirect calorimetry, 5, 223
Infection
  bacterial, 194–197, 202–203
  from catheters, 125, 197, 202
  nosocomial, 202
  tests of, 197–199
Inflammation, 183, 193–197
  applications in patients, 199–201
  bacteria-stimulated events, 195
  chemical products of, 199
  tests of, 197–199
Injury severity score, 225
Inotropes, 38, 39
Interleukin cytokines, 193–194

Intermittent mandatory ventilation (IMV), 80, 81, 90
Interstitial edema, 70, 92–95
Intestinal atrophy, 120, 122
Intracellular fluids, 155, 157

Lactated Ringer's solution, 162
Left ventricular stroke work index, normal value, 30
Lex-O-Con fuel cell system, 9
Life support. *See* Ventilators
Limulus assay, 199
Liver failure, scoring system, 231
Lung dysfunction, 61
Lung volume, 49, 50, 54

Massachusetts General Hospital score, 230
Maximal voluntary ventilation, 111–112
Mechanical ventilation. *See* Ventilators
Mediators, 106, 107
Metabolic rate
  Harris-Benedict equation, 222
  measuring, 101–103
  normal values, 105
Minerals, 108, 124
Mixed expired gas analysis, 2, 3–4
Mixed venous blood (SVO_2), saturation, 18, 60
Monitoring
  cardiac output, 25–27
  electrocardiography, 41–43
  end-tidal CO_2, 66
  oxygenation, 64–65
  saturation, 16–19, 20
Mortality rate
  acute renal failure, 136
  ARF complications, 151
  from exceeding ventilator safe limits, 89
  and nutrition, 112, 129
Motor levels, 179
Multiple-organ failure, 201–204, 226–227
Murray lung score, 230
Myocardial infarction, scoring system, 231

Nephrons, 134
Nephrotoxic agents, 138
Nervous system, 176–181
Neutrophils, 193–194, 197
Nitrogen balance
  determination of, 112
  negative, 107
  vs. energy balance, 118
Nitrogen flux, 107
Nutrition, 102, 103–106
  and acute renal failure, 141–143
  algorithm, 128
  assessment of, 111–113, 126–127
  axioms, 130
  and mortality rate, 112, 129
  nutritional therapy, 117–118
  protein, 107
  vitamins and trace metals, 108, 124

Open wounds, 107, 206–208
Oral tracheal intubation, 78
Osmolality, 217
Oximeters, 8
Oxygen content
  arterial blood, 4, 5–6, 9–10, 16–19, 25
  hemoglobin, 5–6, 7–8
  measuring, 6–9
  pulmonary capillaries, 55, 59–60
  venous blood, 2, 6, 10, 13, 16–19, 57, 63
Oxygen delivery (DO_2), 2, 5–11, 12
  autoregulation, 11, 15–19
  and cardiac function, 25
  normal value, 10
  during respiratory failure, 76
  and survival rate, 20
Oxygen kinetics, 1–20
  normal values, 10
  respiratory gas exchange, 55–61
  supplemental oxygen, 67
Oxyhemoglobin, 5–6, 7–8

Pancreatitis, scoring system, 231
Parenchymal disease, 136–138
Parenteral feeding, 117, 120, 124–125
  electrolytes, 162–164
  formulas, 121, 126
  guidelines, 127

Partial thromboplastin time (PTT), 188, 189, 191
Peritoneal dialysis, 144, 145–146
Pigment nephropathy, 137–138
Plasma, 94, 192
Plasmin, 189
Plateau pressure, 91
Platelets, 187, 190, 191
   activation of, 183, 184–185, 186
   transfusion of, 192
Pneumonia, nosocomial, 203
Pneumotachygraph, 53
Positive end-expiratory pressure (PEEP), 31–32, 52, 71, 73–74
   mechanical ventilation, 79, 80
   during respiratory failure, 73–74, 76, 82
"Pressor" drugs, 39
Pressure support, 90, 91
Pressure-controlled, inverse-ratio ventilation (PCRIV), 89–90
Protein balance, 114–117
"Protein floor," 110
Proteins
   during acute renal failure, 141–142
   catabolic rate, 224
   endogenous sources, 109–113
   exogenous sources, 107
   expenditure with clinical conditions, 102
   in feeding formulas, 119, 124
   metabolism, 106–107
   nutritional therapy, 117
   reserves, 111–113
Protein-sparing effect, 103, 107
Pulmonary artery pressure, 26, 36
   normal value, 30
Pulmonary capillary leakage, 71
Pulmonary compliance, 50–53
Pulmonary edema, 68–74, 92–95, 139
Pulmonary mechanics, 48, 49–53, 56
   effect of position on, 53–55
Pulmonary shunt, 220–221
Pulmonary vascular resistance, 24, 53
   normal value, 30
Pulmonary wedge pressure, 26, 27, 28, 29
   measuring, 31
   normal value, 30, 36
Pulse oximeters, 8
Pus, 194, 195, 206

Quasistatic compliance testing, 52

Rate pressure product, normal value, 30
Renal failure. *See* Acute renal failure (ARF)
Renal physiology, 134–136
Renal replacement therapies, 143–150
Respiratory dead space, 221–222
Respiratory failure, 48, 54, 55
   alarms, 95
   management, 74–77. *See also* Ventilators
   mechanical causes, 74
   pathophysiology, 65–74
   severe, 82–83, 89–95
   ventilators, 89–95
Respiratory physiology
   definitions, 48
   normal values, 56
Respiratory quotient (RQ), 4
Respiratory therapists, 88
Resting energy expenditure (REE), 10, 101
   changes with clinical conditions, 104, 105
   normal value, 105
   relation to size, 103
Right ventricular stroke work index, normal value, 30

Sargent equation, 224
Saturation monitoring, 16–19
Scoring systems, 225–231
Seizures, 18, 180–181
   algorithm, 180
Shock, 37–38, 202, 231
Shunt fraction, 58, 59, 64, 70, 220
Skin test reactivity, 198
Slow continuous ultrafiltration (SCUF), 149–150
Spectrophotometry, 7–8, 62
Spinal cord levels, 178, 179

Spirometry, 2–3, 49, 113
Spontaneous breathing with intermittent mandatory ventilation (SIMV), 80, 81, 90
Starvation, 109–110, 164
  adaptation, 104
Static compliance measurement, 52
Stress ulceration, 122–123
Stroke index, normal value, 30
Stroke volume, 30
Survival rate, 20
  acute renal failure, 150–151
  and nutrition, 129
Swan-Ganz catheter, 31
Synchronized intermittent mandatory ventilation, 81
Systemic inflammatory response syndrome (SIRS), 197, 201–204, 227
Systemic vascular resistance, 24, 35–36

Temperature correction factors, 216
Third-space loss, 156, 157–158
Thrombopoietin, 187
Thrombosis, 183, 184, 187–189
Trace metals, 108, 124
Tracheostomy, 78
Trauma, 181, 225–226
Trauma/injury severity score (TRISS), 225
Tropocollagen, 204

Van Slyke method, 8–9
Venous oxygen content. *See* Oxygen content, venous blood
Ventilation, 80, 90
Ventilation-perfusion (V/Q) matching, 49, 57, 58, 60
  during alveolar collapse, 66
  during pulmonary edema, 68, 69
Ventilators, 52–53, 78
  CO_2 regulation, 77
  controls, 79–80
  learning to manage, 87–88
  management, 79–87
  safe limits, 89
  in severe respiratory failure, 82–83, 89–95
  weaning parameters, 83–87
Vitamins, 108, 124
Volume
  blood, 24–45, 155–156
  lung, 49, 50, 54
  stroke, 30
Volume-assured pressure support (VAPS), 91
von Willebrand factor, 184, 186

Water
  body composition, 155–157
  and electrolyte balance, 159–161
  requirements, 167
Weaning, from mechanical ventilation, 83–87
Wounds, open, 107, 206–208

Made in the USA
Middletown, DE
22 June 2020